AF289877

The Role of Lymphocytes and Macrophages in the Immunological Response

XIII International Congress of Haematology, Munich
August 2—8, 1970

Edited by D. C. Dumonde

With 37 Figures

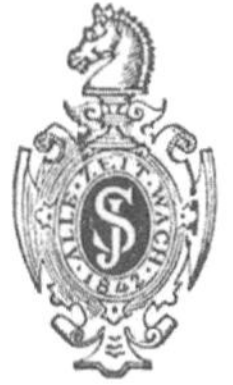

Springer-Verlag
Berlin · Heidelberg · New York 1971

Dr. Dudley Cohen Dumonde, Kennedy Institute of Rheumatology,
Division of Immunology, Bute Gardens, Hammersmith, London, W 6/Great Britain

ISBN-13: 978-3-642-65135-9   e-ISBN-13: 978-3-642-65133-5
DOI: 10.1007/978-3-642-65133-5

Preface: Editorial Introduction

This volume contains papers presented at a symposium on "The Role of Lymphocytes and Macrophages in the Immunological Response" at the XIII International Congress of Haematology, Munich, August 1970.

This symposium was designed to highlight current work submitted to the Haematology Congress which related to the role of cellular cooperation in induction and expression of the immune response. The symposium was divided into two parts. The morning session consisted of invited papers dealing with various general aspects of the field (papers 1 to 5) which were relevant to the afternoon session, which consisted of free communications submitted to the Congress.

In the discussion it was emphasized that whereas lymphocyte activity ultimately underlies all immune induction, the cellular and humoral manifestations of the immune response are governed by distinct yet interacting compartments of the lymphoid system. Much interest centred on the role of thymus-derived lymphocytes as cooperator cells in antibody formation; and the mechanisms by which macrophages assist antibody production. The discussion brought together work on lymphocyte activation, the generation of lymphocyte activation products (lymphokine factors) and the cellular events underlying the induction and expression of the immune response.

The helpful cooperation of Springer-Verlag has enabled rapid publication of the papers presented at this symposium.

London, February 1971

D. C. DUMONDE
Symposium Moderator

Contents

Author Index

D. C. Dumonde, Division of Immunology, Kennedy Institute of Rheumatology, *Hammersmith, London W 6/Great Britain*

D. J. Anstee, Bristol Regional Blood Transfusion Service, *Southmead, Bristol/Great Britain*

G. Alzer, Medizinische Universitätsklinik, *D-5000 Köln-Lindenthal*

H. Asamer, Medizinische Universitätsklinik, *Innsbruck/Austria*

G. W. G. Bird, Birmingham Regional Blood Transfusion Service, *Birmingham 15/ Great Britain*

P. Byrt, The Walter and Eliza Hall Institute of Medical Research, Royal Melbourne Hospital, *Parkville 3050, Australia*

M. J. Cline, University of California, *San Francisco, CA 94122/USA*

P. Drings, Medizinische Universitätsklinik, *D-6900 Heidelberg*

H. M. Dosch, Medizinische Klinik der Universität, *D-355 Marburg*

S. D. Douglas, Mount Sinai School of Medicine, *New York, NY 10029/USA*

H.-D. Flad, Abteilung für klinische Physiologie des Zentrums für klinische Grundlagenforschung der Universität Ulm, *D-7900 Ulm/Donau*, Parkstraße 11

M. Fukase, The Second Division of Department of Internal Medicine, Faculty of Medicine, Kyoto University, *Kyoto/Japan*

R. Gross, Medizinische Universitätsklinik, *D-5000 Köln-Lindenthal*

K. U. Hartmann, Max-Planck-Institut für Virusforschung, Abteilung Physikalische Biologie, *D-7400 Tübingen*

K. Havemann, Medizinische Klinik der Universität, *D-355 Marburg*

W. D. Hirschmann, Medizinische Universitätsklinik, *D-5000 Köln-Lindenthal*

G. Hochapfel, Abteilung für klinische Physiologie des Zentrums für klinische Grundlagenforschung der Universität Ulm, *D-7900 Ulm/Donau*, Parkstraße 11

T. Hoshino, The Second Division of Department of Internal Medicine, Faculty of Medicine, Kyoto University, *Kyoto/Japan*

C. Huber, Medizinische Universitätsklinik, *Innsbruck/Austria*

H. Huber, Medizinische Universitätsklinik, *Innsbruck/Austria*

S. Itani, The Second Division of Department of Internal Medicine, Faculty of Medicine, Kyoto University, *Kyoto/Japan*

D. Jacherts, Institut für Hygiene und Medizinische Mikrobiologie, *CH-3000 Bern,* Friedbühlstraße 51

S. Kawasaki, The Second Division of Department of Internal Medicine, Faculty of Medicine, Kyoto University, *Kyoto/Japan*

E. Leuchars, Chester Beatty Research Institute, Institute of Cancer Research, Royal Cancer Hospital, *Fulham Road, London, S.W.3/Great Britain*

R. N. Maini, Division of Clinical Research, Kennedy Institute of Rheumatology, *Hammersmith, London W 6/Great Britain*

H. Malchow, Medizinische Klinik der Universität, *D-355 Marburg*

T. Mandel, The Walter and Eliza Hall Institute of Medical Research, Royal Melbourne Hospital, *Parkville 3050, Australia*

M. Matthew, Division of Immunology, Kennedy Institute of Rheumatology, *Hammersmith, London W 6/Great Britain*

G. Michlmayr, Medizinische Universitätsklinik, *Innsbruck/Austria*

S. Nakayama, The Second Division of Department of Internal Medicine, Faculty of Medicine, Kyoto University, *Kyoto/Japan*

C. Oates, Division of Immunology, Kennedy Institute of Rheumatology, *Hammersmith, London W 6/Great Britain*

H. Oerkermann, Medizinische Universitätsklinik, *D-5000 Köln-Lindenthal*

G. I. Pardoe, Department of Experimental Pathology, Medical School, University of Birmingham, *Birmingham 15/Great Britain*

P. G. Rigby, University of Nebraska, College of Medicine, *Omaha, NB 68105/USA*

G. E. Roelants, National Institute for Medical Research, *Mill Hill, London NW 7/ Great Britain*

M. Schmidt, Medizinische Klinik der Universität, *D-355 Marburg*

K. Schumacher, Medizinische Universitätsklinik, *D-5000 Köln-Lindenthal*

M. R. Schwarz, Department of Biological Structure, University of Washington, *Seattle, WA 98105/USA*

C. P. Sodomann, Medizinische Klinik der Universität, *D-355 Marburg*

G. Uhlenbruck, Medizinische Universitätsklinik, *D-5000 Köln-Lindenthal*

G. Wintzer, Medizinische Universitätsklinik, *D-5000 Köln-Lindenthal*

R. A. Wolstencroft, Division of Immunology, Kennedy Institute of Rheumatology, *Hammersmith, London W 6/Great Britain*

The Spectrum of Thymus Dependency

E. Leuchars

Introduction

Studies on the thymus have revealed differences in its control of the development of immunological responsiveness in different species [1]. In the chicken, cell-mediated immune responses have been demonstrated to be thymus-dependent but humoral antibody responses have been found to be affected by a different lymphoid organ, the bursa of Fabricius [2]. It has been argued that a similar system might operate in mammals [3, 4] but investigations in the mouse have so far failed to reveal unequivocal evidence of a dichotomy in the development of immunological responsiveness. Studying the responses to a wide variety of antigens, varying from skin homografts and oxazolone to serum proteins and bacterial antigens, in normal, thymus-deprived and thymus-reconstituted CBA mice, it has been show that all, with the possible exception of pneumococcal polysaccharide, are thymus dependent. This finding will be considered in relation to the numbers of residual thymus-derived cells in deprived mice [5]. The significance of the demonstrated spectrum of thymus dependency in mice and its relation to the "bursal equivalent" theory will be discussed.

Experimental Procedure

A variety of responses have been tested using a standard experimental system. Details of this system have been described previously [6] but an outline of the method of preparation of the test mice is shown in Table 1. Bone marrow cells and thymus grafts were given on the day of irradiation. Mice were tested with the appropriate stimulus approximately 50 days later.

Table 1. *Groups of CBA/Lac male mice used to test the thymus dependency of various responses*

Group	Thymus *in situ*	Irradiation (850 r)	Bone marrow (5×10^6 syngeneic cells I.V.)	Thymus graft (1 syngeneic neonatal thymus lobe under kidney capsule)
Normal	+	—	—	—
Deprived	—	+	+	—
Reconstituted	—	+	+	+

Results

The results which have been obtained are summarised in Table 2. The extent to which each response depended on the presence of thymus tissue is indicated.

Table 2. *Thymus dependency of a variety of responses*

Test material	Response measured	Thymus dependent or not	Reference
In vivo:			
Oxazolone	Contact sensitivity	+	7
			8
Skin homograft	Rejection	+	9
Tumour homograft	Control of growth	+	10
Sheep red blood cells	Haemagglutinin and haemolysin titres	+	11
Maia squinada haemocyanin	Antibody titre (antigen binding capacity)	+	12
NIP-BSA	Antibody titre (modified phage inactivation)	+	13
Bacteriophage fd	Antibody titre (phage inactivation)	+	14
Salmonellar flagellar antigen	Agglutinin titre	±	15
Pneumococcal polysaccharide	Agglutinin titre	? —	15
Leishmania tropica promastigotes (ID)	Healing of lesion	+	16
Trichinella spiralis larvae(IV)	Eosinophil count	+	17
Experimentally induced pyelonephritis	Neutrophil count	—	17
In vitro:			
PHA	Lymphocyte transformation	+	5

Discussion

The majority of the responses reviewed in Table 2 have proved to be thymus-dependent. However, the mechanism by which the thymus exerts an effect in such a wide range of reactions is by no means fully understood.

Of the responses listed above, the ability to make antibody to sheep red blood cells has been most fully investigated [6, 18, 19, 20]. It has been shown that the thymus provides cells, "T lymphocytes" [21], which are essential for the full expression of the antibody response. These cells react by mitosis to antigen [6] but are not the cells which secrete antibody [7]. The cells which co-operate with "T lymphocytes" and give rise to plasma cells have been called "B lymphocytes" [21] to indicate that they may be "bursal-equivalent cells"; but there is as yet no critical evidence that a "bursal-equivalent" exists in mammals, although gut-associated lymphoid tissue, or one of its components, has been widely quoted as the most likely candidate [4, 22, 23, 24].

It seems probable that after birth all lymphocytes or their precursors originate in the bone marrow and there is evidence that cells of marrow origin can migrate into the thymus [25] where they undergo a process of differentiation and subsequently emerge [26]. At present we have no evidence that a similar processing of bone-marrow derived cells occurs within the gut-associated lymphoid tissue, nor that the latter is substantially different from the rest of the peripheral lymphoid tissue [27]. Lymphocytes which colonize the peripheral lymphoid organs and give rise to the effector cells in antibody production could already be mature when they emerge from the bone marrow.

Lymphoid cell co-operation has also been demonstrated in the production of anti-BSA antibodies [28], in the response to hapten-carrier conjugates [29, 30] and in graft-versus-host reactions [31, 32]. To what extent such co-operation occurs in other responses, and in particular in delayed hypersensitivity responses and in homograft rejections is not clear, nor is it known whether a similar phenomenon occurs in other species. However, if cell co-operation occurs in the chicken it could explain why delayed hypersensitivity reactions appeared to be dependent on a functioning bursa and also why neither cells from bursectomized nor from thymectomized chickens were on their own able to mount a graft-versus-host attack [2].

In conclusion it may be said that in mammals there is a thymus-dependent component both in cell-mediated immunity and in humoral immunity, at least as regards the production of 7S IgG antibodies. Whether or not the production of 19S IgM antibodies is also thymus-dependent is more questionable. It is interesting to speculate that only small numbers of "T cells" may be required for the production of these antibodies (which may be the only class of antibody being produced in response to pneumococcal polysaccharide [15]) and that sufficient numbers are present in our deprived mice [5] for this component of the response to be potentiated. Elucidation of this point, and indeed the whole question of whether any immune response or any part of it can be said be totally thymus-independent rests on our ability to lower and possibly eventually obliterate this background of "T cells". Perhaps tests on the mutant "nu nu" mice [33], experimental models with congenital aplasia of the thymus, will give us an answer.

Acknowledgements

The work carried out at the Chester Beatty Research Institute (Institute of Cancer Research: Royal Cancer Hospital) was supported by grants from the Medical Research Council and the Cancer Research Campaign.

References

1. MILLER, J. F. A. P., OSOBA, D.: Physiol. Rev. 47, 437 (1967).
2. WARNER, N. L., SZENBERG, A., in: The Thymus in Immunobiology. Eds.: R. A. GOOD and A. E. GABRIELSON. New York: Harper and Row 1964, p. 395.
3. COOPER, M. D., PETERSON, R. D. A., GOOD, R. A.: Nature (Lond.) 205, 143 (1965).
4. — PEREY, D. Y., McKNEALLY, M. F., GABRIELSON, A. E., SUTHERLAND, D. E., GOOD, R. A.: Lancet 1966 I, 1388.

5. DOENHOFF, M. J., DAVIES, A. J. S., LEUCHARS, E., WALLIS, V.: Proc. roy. Soc. B., **176**, 69 (1970).
6. DAVIES, A. J. S., LEUCHARS, E., WALLIS, V., KOLLER, P. C.: Transplantation **4**, 438 (1966).
7. — CARTER, R. L., LEUCHARS, E., WALLIS, V.: Immunology **17**, 111 (1969).
8. PARROTT, D. M. V., DE SOUSA, M. A. B., FACHET, J., WALLIS, V., LEUCHARS, E., DAVIES, A. J. S.: Clin. exp. Immunol. **7**, 387 (1970).
9. LEUCHARS, E., CROSS, A. M., DUKOR, P.: Transplantation **3**, 28 (1965).
10. WESTON, B.: Unpublished observations (1970).
11. DAVIES, A. J. S., CARTER, R. L., LEUCHARS, E., WALLIS, V., KOLLER, P. C.: Immunology **16**, 57 (1969).
12. ASKONAS, B. A.: Unpublished observations (1970).
13. AIRD, J.: Immunology. In press (1971).
14. KOLSCH, E.: In press (1970).
15. DAVIES, A. J. S., CARTER, R. L., LEUCHARS, E., WALLIS, V., DIETRICH, F. M.: Immunology **19**, 745 (1970).
16. PRESTON, P., DUMONDE, D. C.: Unpublished observations (1970).
17. WALLS, R. S., BASTEN, A.: Unpublished observations (1970).
18. CLAMAN, H. N., CHAPERON, E. A., TRIPLETT, R. F.: J. Immunol. **97**, 828 (1966).
19. DAVIES, A. J. S., LEUCHARS, E., WALLIS, V., MARCHANT, R., ELLIOT, E V.: Transplantation **5**, 222 (1967).
20. MITCHELL, G. F., MILLER, J. F. A. P.: J. exp. Med. **128**, 821 (1968).
21. ROITT, I. M., GREAVES, M. F., TORRIGIANI, G., BROSTOFF, J., PLAYFAIR, J. H. L.: Lancet 1969 II, 367.
22. ARCHER, O. K., SUTHERLAND, D. E. R., GOOD, R. A.: Nature (Lond.) **200**, 337 (1963).
23. FICHTELIUS, K. E., YUNIS, E. J., GOOD, R. A.: Proc. Soc. exp. Biol. (N.Y.) **128**, 185 (1968).
24. MEUWISSEN, H. J., KAPLAN, G. T., PEREY, D. Y., GOOD, R. A.: Proc. Soc. exp. Biol. (N.Y.) **130**, 300 (1969).
25. MICKLEM, H. S., FORD, C. E., EVANS, E. P., GRAY, J.: Proc. roy. Soc. B. **165**, 78 (1966).
26. WEISSMAN, I. L.: J. exp. Med. **126**, 291 (1967).
27. COOPER, G. N., THONARD, J. C., CROSBY, R. L., DALBOW, M. H.: Aust. J. exp. Biol. med. Sci. **46**, 407 (1968).
28. TAYLOR, R. B.: Transplant. Rev. **1**, 114 (1969).
29. MITCHISON, N. A., in: Immunological Tolerance. Eds.: Landy and Braun 1969, p. 149.
30. RAFF, M. C.: Nature (Lond.) **226**, 1257 (1970).
31. CANTOR, H., ASOFSKY, R.: J. exp. Med. **131**, 235 (1970).
32. BARCHILON, J., GERSHON, R. K.: Nature (Lond.) **227**, 71 (1970).
33. DE SOUSA, M. A. B., PARROTT, D. M. V., PANTELOURIS, E. M.: Clin. exp. Immunol. **4**, 637 (1969).

The Flow of Information during Primary Antibody Synthesis

D. JACHERTS

With 3 Figures

Antibody synthesis has been compared by several authors with enzyme induction [2—5]. This comparison is in contrast to the conceptions of the selective theory [6—8] and its modifications [9, 10] which regard antibody synthesis as a constitutional activity of single cells, the increase of antibody following contact with an antigen being thought to be a problem of population genetics. At least, since the induction of β-galactosidase synthesis in E. coli has been clarified, the conception of antibody synthesis as an enzyme induction constitutes an alternative to the instructive theories [11—14]. With increasing knowledge of protein synthesis, it had to be expected that analogies would be found between antibody synthesis and any other protein synthesis when the discussion is limited to the events occurring on ribosomes. In attempting to summarize clearly recognizable differences between an inducible protein synthesis and antibody synthesis, the following should be noted predominantly:

1. Two cell types are involved in antibody synthesis [15—18]. Primary antigen receptors recognize antigens as such and subsequently produce RNA which is transferred to other cells able to produce antibodies. It is in these cells that the humoral antibodies are synthesized.

2. While inducible enzymes are usually homogeneous proteins, antibodies are of considerable diversity [19]. This diversity concerns not only the amount of energy of the antigen-antibody binding but also the molecular configuration of antibodies, as can be seen in the different classes (IgG, IgA, etc.) and allotypes.

Because of these essential features of antibody synthesis, it is not easy to compare antibody synthesis with enzyme induction. The prerequisite of interaction between antigen-recognizing and antibody-producing cells involves a special transfer of information. Since this transfer of information was not yet known in cells of macroorganisms, it seems reasonable to describe this flow of information during antibody synthesis. FISHMAN [15] and MITSUHASHI et al. [16] were the first to show that macrophages synthesize an RNA after contact with antigen and that this RNA initiates antibody synthesis after being transferred to lymphoid cells. Other authors claimed that this RNA was contaminated with antigen [19—22]. Therefore, the first problem which raises is the question concerning the content of information of this RNA and the importance of possible antigenic impurities. FISHMAN [23] established this RNA as the sole carrier of information by proving synthesis of donor-specific antibodies in an allotypically defined animal. SAITO et al. excluded an informative activity of the antigen by serial dilutions of RNA in experimental animals [24].

Our own experiments differ in two essential points from the ones mentioned above. At first, we attempted to determine the optimal doses of antigen [25, 26]. Optimal doses refer to those which are able to induce RNA synthesis and synthesis of immunologically specific proteins in the shortest time possible. It ranges about 6 to 9 orders of magnitude below the antigen doses used by the authors mentioned above. Furthermore, we not only examined the information of this RNA in animals and cell cultures but also in a cell-free system [27, 28].

As far as function is concerned, our results are analogous to those obtained by FISHMAN and MITSUHASHI et al. Chemically our own RNA differs from the preparations of these authors. Characteristic features are: density in CsCl 1.881, in Cs_3SO_4 1.67, heat stability at 100° C and an extremely high RNase-sensitivity. The informative RNA (i-RNA) seems to be a single-stranded RNA molecule. As can be seen from Fig. 1, this i-RNA has possibly a special configuration which is responsible for its

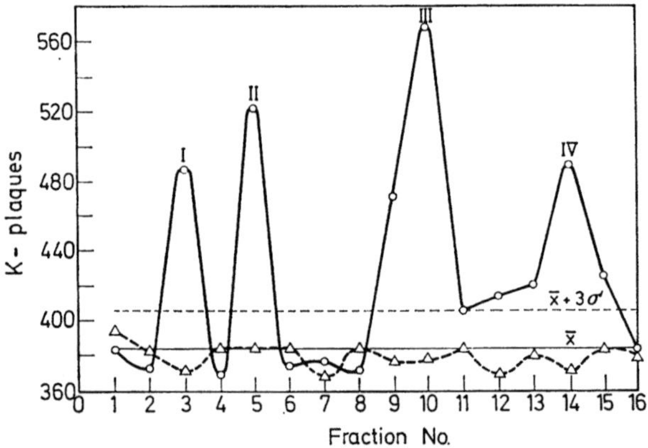

Fig. 1. Biological activity of i-RNA$_{Rk}$ after sedimentation through a sucrose gradient, ranging from 5—25⁰/o sucrose, 100,000 g, 2ʰ. Each fraction was incubated with the protein-synthesizing cell-free system (pH 5 fraction and ribosomes) for synthesis of antibodies against the phage receptor particle R_k. Antibody is estimated by receptor neutralisation. O ——— O i-RNA$_{Rk}$ isolated from a cell-free system which has been stimulated with the phage receptor particle R_k as antigen; △————△ control RNA isolated from a nonstimulated cell-free system

high sedimentation coefficients, ranging from 240 in fraction I to 19 in fraction IV. In allotypically heterologous cell-free systems it is capable of expressing the allotype of the donor on the antibody (Table 1). It can induce antibody synthesis in intact hosts (Table 2). I should be kept in mind that we are able to induce antibody synthesis with RNA doses several orders of magnitude lower than those of other authors and that there is no simple relationship between the amount of antibody synthesized and the RNA doses applied. Of special interest is the observation that antibody synthesis is not induced by application of higher doses of informative

RNA or several single doses of i-RNA. The i-RNA is synthesized on the DNA of the primary antigen-accepting cell [29]. The primary antigen-accepting cell is multipotent as regards recognizable antigens [28] and for each immunological specificity a distinct gene exists on the DNA.

Table 1

Allotypes		
of the donor of DNA from which i-RNA has been transcribed after antigenic stimulation	of the cell-free system in which the i-RNA has synthesized antibody	of antibody synthesized in the cell-free system
$InV\ 1^+$	$InV\ 1^-$	$InV\ 1^+$
$InV\ 1^-$	$InV\ 1^+$	$InV\ 1^-$
$Gm_{1-4+12+}$	$Gm_{1+4-12-}$	$Gm_{1-4+12+}$
Gm_{2-}	Gm_{2+}	Gm_{2-}
$Gm_{1-}InV\ 1^+$	$Gm_{1+}InV\ 1^-$	$Gm_{1-}InV\ 1^+$
Gm_{1-2-}	Gm_{1+2+}	Gm_{1-2-}

The synthesis of informative RNA can proceed in a cell-free system. Provided optimal concentrations of the reactants are present, the cell-free system is a very favorable experimental set-up for following the flow of information during antibody synthesis. In a cell-free system the synthesis of i-RNA can readily be distinguished from synthesis of antibody. The system for RNA synthesis consists of 10^{-4} µg DNA/ml and of pH 5 fraction at a concentration of 0.3 mg nitrogen/ml. Curiously enough, the optimal concentration of antigen is also very constant. For all antigens tested so far it amounts to 10^6 particles/ml.

In a cell-free system the DNA can derive from any cells within a species, while pH 5 fraction has to be prepared from immunologically competent cells [29]. Therefore, the assumption is justified that the genome of any cell contains the information for antibody synthesis. The comparison of antibody synthesis with enzyme induction seems to be justified in that the genetic information present in all cells can be transcribed into an RNA only by certain definite cells after contact with the antigen. Another cell-free system is suitable for synthesis of antibodies and for testing the biological activity of i-RNA. This system consists of pH 5 fraction at an optimal concentration of 0.3 mg nitrogen/ml, ribosomes from immunocompetent cells (lymphocytes, spleen cells, peripheral leucocytes) at an optimal concentration of $3.0\ 10^{-3}$ µg nitrogen/ml and informative RNA. Since this system does not contain any DNA all information for the synthesis of antibody cames from i-RNA.

Informative RNA can be inactivated by irradiation with UV light or γ rays. In this way it is possible to determine the size of the informatively active site on this RNA by comparing the rate of inactivation of the i-RNA with the rate of inactivation of different single-stranded nucleic acid molecules of known length. So far, this type of experiment has been performed with i-RNA of mice and man. The results are shown in Table 3 [30, 31]. The analysis of the target size shows that sufficient triplets are present on the fractions I, II and III of i-RNA to code for a

Table 2. *Antibody response in guinea pigs to inoculation with graded doses of informational RNA and of control RNA from non-stimulated cell-free systems*

Exper. No.	Primary Inoculation with RNA		Antibody Response to A/1/PR301 [a]										
	Type	Dose of RNA given/ animal	ACU titer [g]								Neutralization titer *in ovo*		
			0 [b]	7 [b]	13 [b]	21 [b]	42 [b]	153 [b]	158 [b]	170 [b]	153 [b]	158 [b]	170 [b]
		µg											
1	Informational RNA [c]	0.535 [d]	<15	750	194	n. t.	1009	103	95	106	<28	79	50
2	Informational RNA [c]	0.053 [d]	<15	<15	<15	<15	<15	n.t.	n.t.	n.t.	n.t.	n.t.	n.t.
3	Informational RNA [c]	0.0053 [d]	<15	280	1026	750	658	n.t.	n.t.	n.t.	n.t.	n.t.	n.t.
4	Informational RNA [c]	0.00053 [d]	<15	1397	450	1800	672	<15	<15	108	<28	<28	<28
5	Control RNA	0.321 [d]	<15	<15	<15	<15	<15	<15	<15	<15	<28	<28	<28
6	Informational RNA [c]	0.0265 [e]	<15	<15	<15	<15	<15	<15	<15	125	<28	<28	39
7	Control RNA	0.0265 [e]	<15	<15	<15	<15	<15	<15	<15	<15	<28	<28	<28
8	Informational RNA [c]	0.0053 [f]	<15	<15	600	1600	500	<15	<15	n.t.	<28	<28	56
9	Control RNA	0.00325 [f]	<15	<15	<15	<15	<15	<15	<15	<15	<28	<28	<28

[a] None of the sera tested showed detectable antibody against A/2/AA/1/65 and B/Belfast/841/61.
[b] Days after primary inoculation.
[c] Obtained by stimulating a cell-free system with hemagglutinins of strains A/1/PR301, A/2/AA/1/65 and B/Belfast/841/61.
[d] Injected in 1 ml subcutaneously.
[e] Injected in five doses (each 30 ml) intraperitoneally.
[f] Injected in 1 ml intraperitoneally.
154 days after first inoculation, each of the animals of groups 1, 4, 6 and 8 was restimulated with 1 ml of informational RNA (0.0093 µg RNA/ml, cell-free system stimulated with A/1/PR301 hemagglutinin) subcutaneously, and each of the animals of groups 5, 7 and 9 received 1 ml "control RNA" (0.0067 µg RNA/ml) subcutaneously.
[g] ACU = Antibody concentration unit (25).

Table 3

RNA fraction	Target size (number of nucleotides) calculated on the basis of		Number of triplets in the informational active region
	γ-irradiation	UV-irradiation	
RNA$_{Rk}$ I [a, c]	$5.1 \cdot 10^3$		$1.7 \cdot 10^3$
RNA$_{R_5}$ I [b]		$4.7 \cdot 10^3$	$1.5 \cdot 10^3$
RNA$_{Rk}$ II		$3.3 \cdot 10^3$	$1.1 \cdot 10^3$
RNA$_{Rk}$ II	$3.6 \cdot 10^3$		$1.2 \cdot 10^3$
RNA$_{R_5}$ II		$2.7 \cdot 10^3$	$9.0 \cdot 10^2$
RNA$_{Rk}$ III		$2.3 \cdot 10^3$	$7.7 \cdot 10^2$
RNA$_{Rk}$ III	$1.8 \cdot 10^3$		$6.0 \cdot 10^2$
RNA$_{R_5}$ III		$2.7 \cdot 10^3$	$9.0 \cdot 10^2$
RNA$_{Rk}$ IV			$2.9 \cdot 10^2$
RNA$_{Rk}$ IV	$8.7 \cdot 10^2$	$1.2 \cdot 10^3$	$4.0 \cdot 10^2$
RNA$_{R_5}$ IV		$1.1 \cdot 10^3$	$3.6 \cdot 10^2$

[a] RNA$_{Rk}$ is an i-RNA which codes for antibody against the phage receptor particle Rk.

[b] RNA$_{R_5}$ is an i-RNA which codes for antibody against the phage receptor particle R_5.

[c] I, II, III and IV are the four biological active i-RNA-fractions from a sucrose gradient (cf. Fig. 1).

complete antibody. The analysis of the target size does not answer the question whether the information for the antibody is compiled on a single RNA molecule, or whether two or more independent RNA molecules are necessary for the synthesis of one antibody molecule. Several authors suggested that heavy and light chains of the antibody are synthesized separately [32—35]. Polysomes for the synthesis of light and polysomes for the synthesis of heavy chains could be demonstrated. Therefore, the information for the synthesis of a complete antibody is distributed among several equally important RNA molecules which convey information during synthesis. Thus, it may be that one kind of RNA molecule codes for the parts reacting with the antigen while another kind directs the synthesis of those parts of the antibody that do not react with the antigen. In this case the activity of an irradiated i-RNA should be restored by addition of a non-irradiated i-RNA which codes for an immunologically different antibody. RNA molecules damaged by UV light and responsible for the synthesis of antibody areas which do not react with the antigen could be replaced by the corresponding undamaged RNA molecules. If, on the other hand, specific as well as non-specific parts of the antibody are coded by the same RNA molecule, the mentioned exchange of RNA molecules should not be possible. If this is true, the addition of a non-irradiated preparation of i-RNA cannot restore the activity of the irradiated RNA. The results of such an experiment are shown in Fig. 2. It can be seen that, in fact, the information for antibody synthesis is distributed between i-RNA molecules which at least can be divided into

two classes: RNA molecules which code for immunological specificity, and
RNA molecules which code for parts of the antibody not reacting with the
antigen. Furthermore, this experiment tests the size of those RNA molecules
which are responsible for the immunological specificity of the antibody. Fig. 2 shows
that about 30⁰/o of the total target size is necessary for the immunological specificity

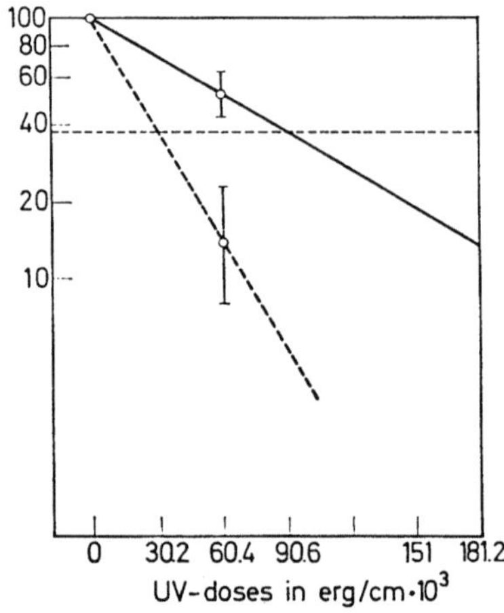

Fig. 2. Inactivation of i-RNA by UV irradiation (— — — —) and rescue of the informative
activity by addition of undamaged i-RNA for synthesis of antibodies of different immunological specificity (————). Bars represent $\bar{x} \pm 3\,\sigma$

of the antibody molecule. This result is unexpected since it corresponds to a part
of the antibody about the size of light chains. However, the heavy chains react
predominantly with an antigen while the light chains are involved in the binding
of the antigen to only a small extent. Assuming that the heavy chain is synthesized in
one piece, the results have to be interpreted as meaning that the i-RNA is not always
present in distinct and equally important subunits for synthesis of the immunologically specific and the non-specific parts, but that it can combine to form a single
molecule which contains the information for the immunologically specific as well
as the non-specific parts of the antibody. This would mean that i-RNA molecules
are able to recombine with one another. If the possibility of recombination of i-RNA
molecules is rejected, it has to be admitted that heavy chains are synthesized in two
or more subunits which subsequently combine to form a larger molecule, that is, the
heavy chain. In both cases the information for the synthesis of heavy chains would
derive from two different molecules. In the first case the recombining reaction would
be expected before synthesis of the heavy chains, whereas in the second case the
recombination should occur after synthesis of the subunits. As far as the problem
of diversity of antibody molecules is concerned, it does no matter whether the
recombination occurs on the level of informative RNA or on the level of hypothetical
subunits of heavy chains.

Spleen cell cultures free of macrophages are not capable of giving a primary
reaction with an antigen. In spleen cell cultures, antibody synthesis occurs only

after addition of i-RNA, reaching its maximum after about one day and persisting usually up to six days. Following this productive phase of antibody synthesis, spleen cell cultures have a latent phase. During this latent phase no i-RNA is detectable by preparative methods, nor is it possible to isolate antibodies from spleen cell cultures during this phase. Nevertheless, the spleen cell culture of the latent phase differs markedly from primary spleen cell cultures before application of i-RNA. At this point it is able to react with the antigen and—after contact with optimal doses of antigen—once more to induce the synthesis of i-RNA and antibodies. It now combines properties which had originally been found in macrophages, that is, recognition of the antigen and subsequent synthesis of i-RNA, with properties which had so far been found only in antibody producers, that is, the synthesis of humoral antibodies.

Even more surprising is the finding that such a spleen cell culture in the latent phase can be induced by non-specific stress to synthesize i-RNA and antibodies, for instance, by UV irradiation. After UV irradiation a striking synthesis of i-RNA can be observed, but this synthesis differs distinctly from primary synthesis of i-RNA in macrophages. Latent cells synthesize i-RNA after UV irradiation in the presence of actinomycin. This means that after UV irradiation the i-RNA is synthesized independently of the genome. In antibody-producing cells, i-RNA can be stored for prolonged periods in the cellular cytoplasm during the latent phase, comparable to a latent virus. Furthermore, in these cells i-RNA can be synthesized on i-RNA [36] independently of the DNA.

The 10^{-4} µg DNA present in the cell-free system corresponds to the amount of DNA present in about 40 cells. Therefore, the gene necessary for a certain synthesis of antibody would be present forty times in the cell-free system. Already after 5 min of incubation with the antigen, at least 100,000 RNA molecules must have been synthesized because otherwise it would not be possible to synthesize antibody after dilution of 10^{-5} in an animal. This means that each genome in the cell-free system is transcribing 2500 RNA molecules per minute. This rate of transcription exceeds any rate of RNA-synthesis so far known.

Immediately after transcription, a mechanism as yet unknown has to initiate the multiplication of i-RNA. Thus, two independent experimental conditions are found which suggest that i-RNA could be replicated on i-RNA.

The ideal starting material for isolating an enzyme which identically replicates i-RNA on i-RNA is the pH 5 fraction. The easiest method for isolation of this replicase is chromatography on Sephadex G 200. The results so far obtained are summarized in Table 4. This shows that it is possible to synthesize i-RNA if replicase, a cofactor and triphosphates are present, provided i-RNA is added to the system as a primer. This system is analogue to that which has been demonstrated in bacteria infected with phages [1, 41]. In addition, the activity of our replicase can be compared to that of bacterial replicase. While the bacterial replicases are strongly specific for the corresponding phage RNA molecules, our replicase is specific for the replication of i-RNA [37—40].

Thus up to this point, the first step in the synthesis of i-RNA corresponds to reactions which are known from enzyme induction. The two possibilities during the next step, that is recombination of i-RNA molecules, and replication of i-RNA molecules, do not correspond to the so-far-known reactions in enzyme induction.

Table 4

	Replicase for i-RNA	Replicase for phage	
		AUGUST	SPIEGELMAN
Sample volume (M)	0,5	0,35	0,25
Triphosphates (M)	10^{-9}	10^{-7}	$2 \cdot 10^{-7}$
Cofactor (μg)	$\sim 10^{-2}$	2—12	—
i-RNA (μg)	$5 \cdot 10^{-2}$	$5 \cdot 10^{-3}$	1
Replicase (μg)	$9 \cdot 10^{-2}$	1—3	50
Incorporated triphosphates (M) per mg protein of enzyme fraction	$2,25 \cdot 10^{-7}$	$1,24 \cdot 10^{-6}$	$4 \cdot 10^{-8}$

Table 5

	Allotypes	
of i-RNA	of the cells in culture	of the antibody synthesized with i-RNA isolated from the cell culture
	Without puromycin	
RNS I Gm 4^+12^+InV 1^+	Gm 4^-12^-InV 1^-	RNS I Gm 4^-12^-InV 1^-
	With puromycin	
RNS I Gm 4^+12^+InV 1^+	Gm 4^-12^-InV 1^-	RNS I Gm 4^+12^+InV 1^+

Rather it is analogous to the physiology of viral nucleic acids and should be—according to known recombinative and replicative processes—an essential cause of the diversity of antibody molecules. Since the discussed results indicate that both replication and recombination of i-RNA molecules are frequent events compared to *de novo* synthesis of i-RNA on the genome, they would be expected to increase the diversity of antibodies immensely. Since previous experience shows that this is not the case, it should be expected that there are feedback mechanisms which from time to time or constantly allow *de novo* synthesis of i-RNA molecules on the genome, thus limiting the diversity of antibody molecules.

If an RNA, which has been transcribed on DNA of allotypically heterologous cells, is added to a cell culture, allotypically heterologous antibodies are initially synthesized by this cell culture. After some time, however, antibodies appear which correspond to the cell culture as far as allotype is concerned. This result shows that antibody synthesis in the cells changes from individually specific heterologous to individually specific homologous antibodies. This switch mechanism can be clarified by separating antibody synthesis from synthesis of i-RNA. In cell cultures, this can be achieved by inhibition of antibody synthesis with puromycin. As Table 5 shows, no

RNA is produced on the genome of antibody-producing cells in the presence of puromycin. The change of allotype does not occur because obviously i-RNA does not synthesize a protein which is necessary for the *de novo* synthesis of i-RNA on the cellular genome. It is much easier to separate antibody synthesis and RNA synthesis in cell-free systems. If pH 5 fraction and ribosomes are present in the system, i-RNA synthesizes protein. These proteins can be fractionated by a sucrose gradient and it can be determined whether they contain antibody activity and a protein which, in its capacity as regulator protein, will initiate RNA synthesis in a second cell-free system, consisting of DNA + pH 5 fraction. As may be seen in Fig. 3, there are, in fact, not only fractions containing antibodies but also fractions containing regulator protein. This protein is the basis for a feedback mechanism which allows *de novo* synthesis of i-RNA on the cellular genome.

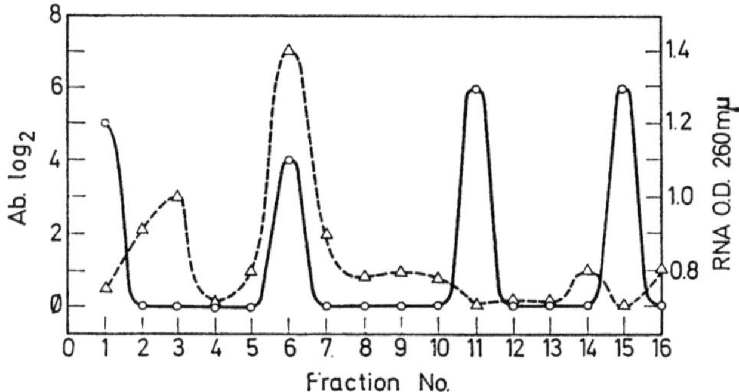

Fig. 3. Separation of antibody activity from regulatory activity by sedimentation through a sucrose gradient (5—25⁰/₀ sucrose, 100.000 g, 15ʰ). △—————△ regulatory activity; ○————————○ antibody activity

The most important results can be summarized as follows:

1. In the primary reaction with an antigen the i-RNA is synthesized on the DNA of an antigen recognizing cell.

2. The i-RNA can be present in subunits which are able to recombine with one another.

3. i-RNA can be replicated independently of the genome by *de novo* synthesis of i-RNA in the presence of replicase.

4. Excessive diversity of antibodies is prevented by a feedback mechanism. In this feedback mechanism, a regulator protein initiates synthesis of i-RNA on the genome, which codes for antibodies with corresponding immunological specificity.

References

1. Haruna, J., Spiegelman, S.: Science **150**, 884 (1965).
2. Dienert, F.: Ann. Inst. Pasteur **14**, 139 (1900).
3. Beiser, S. M., et al.: Nature **189**, 659 (1961).
4. Monod, J., in: Cellular and humoral aspects of the hypersensitive states. New York: Hoeber-Harper 1959, p. 528.

5. SZILARD, L.: Proc. nat. Acad. Sci. (Wash.) **46**, 293 (1960).
6. EHRLICH, P.: Proc. roy. Soc. B **66**, 424 (1900).
7. JERNE, N. K.: Proc. nat. Acad. Sci. (Wash.) **41**, 849 (1955).
8. BURNET, F. M., in: The clonal selection theory of immunity. Nashville (Tenn.): Vanderbilt Univ. Press 1959.
9. SMITHIES, O.: Nature **199**, 1231 (1963).
10. DREYER, W. J., et al.: Cold Spr. Harb. Symp. quant. Biol. **32**, 353 (1970).
11. BREINL, F., et al.: Z. physiol. Chem. **192**, 45 (1930).
12. PAULING, L.: J. Amer. Chem. Soc. **62**, 2643 (1940).
13. HAUROWITZ, F.: Nature **205**, 847 (1965).
14. PARDEE, A. B., et al.: J. molec. Biol. **1**, 165 (1959).
15. FISHMAN, M.: J. exp. Med. **114**, 837 (1961).
16. MITSUHASHI, S., et al.: Jap. J. Microbiol. **12**, 261 (1968).
17. FELDMAN, M., et al.: Cold Spr. Harb. Symp. quant. Biol. **32**, 415 (1967).
18. JACHERTS, D., et al.: Z. med. Mikrobiol. u. Immunol. **152**, 112 (1966).
19. ASKONAS, B. A., et al.: Nature **205**, 470 (1965).
20. FRIEDMAN, H. P., et al.: Science **149**, 1106 (1965).
21. GOTTLIEB, A. A., et al.: Proc. nat. Acad. Sci. (Wash.) **57**, 1849 (1967).
22. ADLER, F. L., et al.: J. Immunol. **97**, 554 (1966).
23. SAITO, K., et al.: Jap. J. Microbiol. **13**, 122 (1969).
24. JACHERTS, D.: Z. med. Microbiol. u. Immunol. **152**, 20 (1966).
25. DRESCHER, J., et al.: Zbl. Bakt., I. Abt. Orig. **199**, 315 (1966).
26. JACHERTS, D.: Z. med. Microbiol. u. Immunol. **154**, 245 (1968).
27. — et al.: J. Immunol. **104**, 746 (1970).
28. — et al.: Z. med. Microbiol. u. Immunol. **152**, 33 (1966).
29. — Z. med. Mikrobiol. u. Immunol. **154**, 300 (1969).
30. — Z. med. Mikrobiol. u. Immunol. **153**, 250 (1967).
31. SCHWEYM, U.: Thesis Techn. Univ. Hannover (1970).
32. SHAPIRO, A., et al.: Proc. nat. Acad. Sci. (Wash.) **56**, 216 (1966).
33. DE PETRIS, S.: J. molec. Biol. **23**, 215 (1967).
34. LA VIA, M. F., et al.: Proc. nat. Acad. Sci. (Wash.) **57**, 79 (1968).
35. NAKASHIMA, S., et al.: Biochim. biophys. Acta (Amst.) **145**, 671 (1967).
36. JACHERTS, D.: Z. med. Mikrobiol. u. Immunol. **152**, 262 (1966).
37. NEUHOFF, V., et al.: Hoppe-Seylers Z. physiol. Chem. **351**, 157 (1970).
38. JACHERTS, D.: Hoppe-Seylers Z. physiol. Chem. **350**, 1162 (1969).
39. — Europ. J. Immunol. Proc. of a Symp. (1969).
40. OPITZ, G.: Thesis Techn. Univ. Hannover (1970).
41. FRANZE, M. T. DE FERNANDEZ, EOYANG, L., AUGUST, J. T.: Nature **219**, 588 (1968).

Biochemical Evidence against a Physiological Role for Macrophage RNA-Antigen Complexes in the Immune Induction

G. E. ROELANTS

In the past few years the concept of cooperation between cells for the induction of an immune response has been well established. It is generally believed that three cells are involved in the process: a lymphoid cell derived from the bone marrow, another lymphoid cell also derived from the bone marrow but "influenced" by the thymus, and a phagocytic cell: the macrophage. The thymus-bone marrow cells interaction is discussed in detail elsewhere in this symposium. Briefly, the "thymus derived" cell plays a role in recognising the antigen but does not secrete antibody. The "bone marrow derived cell" secretes antibody but needs the help of the "thymus derived cell" to do so.

The role left to the phagocytic cell is not clear. Does it merely remove the excess antigen or does it play a more active specific role? We will devote this presentation to the analysis of a theory which stirred up a lot of excitement.

It has been postulated that, after phagocytosis by macrophages, antigens are broken down and that fragments of antigens become associated with RNA. The antigen-RNA complexes would then be transferred to the antibody-forming cell precursor to trigger cell proliferation and antibody production directed against a specific antigenic determinant: the fragment of antigen associated with the RNA.

This concept was first based on the finding that crude filtrates of peritoneal exudate (P. E.) cells exposed to T2 bacteriophages, when incubated with lymph node cells *in vitro,* induced in some cases the production of anti T2 antibody and that this phenomenon was inhibited by ribonuclease treatment of the extract [1]. Subsequent experiments showed that similar results could be obtained using RNA preparations from P. E. cells instead of whole filtrates [2]. The presence of antigen was later demonstrated in similar RNA preparations using the same antigen, T2 phage [3] or *Maia squinada hemocyanin* [4]. With this last molecule the amount of antigen calculated to be present on the immunogenic RNA preparation on the basis of radioactivity was about 20 to 30 times less than the minimum amount of free hemocyanin eliciting a response in mice. Thus, the association with RNA seemed to enhance the immunogenicity of the antigen.

GOTTLIEB et al. [5] after incubation of P. E. cells with T2 bacteriophages assayed activity of RNA fractions on splenic fragments. Low levels of T2 inhibition could be induced by the 28S fraction from sucrose density gradients; the activity persisted after degradation of the RNA to 4-6S fragments. Incorporation of ^{3}H-uridine showed that only 4-5S RNA had been newly synthesized during the time of incubation of P. E. cells with T2 phage.

By DNA hybridization experiments, it was shown that RNA from P. E. cells not exposed to T2 phage [5] or exposed to R17 phage [6] competed for annealing with that of cells exposed to T2. Those results indicate that activity resides in a pre-existing RNA fraction rather than in RNA synthesized following exposure to antigen. When examined in cesium sulfate equilibrium gradients [5], the bulk of the P. E. cells RNA showed a density around 1.665. A minor component, consisting of about 5⁰/o of the total RNA with a density of 1.588, accounted for the total immunogenic activity of the preparation. Its formation was not impaired by actinomycin D. After incubation with antigen it contained antigenic fragments of low molecular weight [8]. When RNA was extracted from P. E. cells which had not been incubated with antigen, the "minor band" also appeared and contained protein [5].

From these observations it was concluded that the "minor band" observed in cesium sulfate consisted of an antigen-RNA complex which "may be the essential means by which the information eliciting specific antibody production is processed, even though the RNA itself is not specific" [5].

Thus, in the above experiments it was clear that, in some cases, an immune response could be induced by antigen-P. E. RNA complexes and, in addition, some of the complexes were partially characterized. Yet it seemed to us that the crucial argument for or against the hypothesis was not to show that a material obtained by breaking up macrophages was immunogenic but to demonstrate that this material, that is antigen-RNA complexes, was indeed formed in intact cells and transferred *in vivo* to the antibody-forming cell precursor.

In this context, one interesting finding was that, in Askonas and Rhodes' experiments with hemocyanin, when RNA was extracted immediately after the addition of ^{131}I-hemocyanin to P. E. cells, that is before any "processing" of the antigen could take place, an RNA containing macromolecular ^{131}I-labelled material could also be obtained and was immunogenic [4]. To try to determine if macrophage RNA-antigen binding was a physiological phenomenon or rather an interesting artefact we decided to examine the following facets of the association:

1. the relationship between molecular structure, immunopotency and capacity to form complexes with RNA.

2. the kinetics of association.

3. the specificity of association.

4. the nature of the chemical bound between antigen and RNA.

The experiments I shall discuss were done in collaboration with Dr. J. W. GOODMAN and have been reported in detail [9, 10]. These observations were also summarized elsewhere [11].

The Relationship between Immunogenicity and Association with RNA

We argued that if the macrophage was the cell responsible for "antigen recognition" and if the formation of macrophage RNA-antigen complexes had an important role in immune induction, there would be some degree of differentiation between molecules on the basis of immunogenicity in the binding process. In the simplest hypothesis good immunogens would associate better with RNA than weak ones and nonimmunogenic molecules would not bind at all. To test this point different compounds including natural and synthetic polypeptides, a protein, polysaccharides, amino acids and steroid hormones were assayed for their capacity to form complexes with P. E. cells RNA (Table 1) [9, 10].

Table 1. *The association of various molecules with RNA from peritoneal exudate cells.* (ROELANTS and GOODMAN, 1969; reprinted with permission from the J. exp. Med.)

Molecule	Total dose range		No. of experiments	Efficiency of binding [a]
	μg	μc		
^{3}H-Poly-γ-D-glutamic acid [b]	40—550	(2.04—28.05)	44 [c]	$1.7—10 \times 10^{-4}$
^{3}H-Poly-α-D-glutamic acid	110—550	16.17—80.85	4	$1.8—4.0 \times 10^{-4}$
^{14}COOH-dextran	572—11450	0.49— 9.96	20	$1.3—4.9 \times 10^{-4}$
^{3}H-Dextran	260	24.96	2	Below detection
^{125}I-Myeloma protein	40	1.62	2	4.7×10^{-5}
^{125}I-(TGAL)	4	8.72	4 [d]	5.0×10^{-5}
^{14}C-Testosterone	10	1.75	2	Below detection
^{3}H-Estradiol	10 [e]	14.68	2	Below detection
^{3}H-Cortisone	10 [e]	9.54	2	Below detection
^{14}C-DL-Glutamic acid	75	3.42	2	4.0×10^{-5}
^{14}C-L-Glutamic acid	75	111.22	2	4.0×10^{-5}

[a] Micrograms of "antigen" complexed per microgram of RNA per microgram of total antigen (intracellular or in homogenate). Corrected for controls (antigen and purified RNA mixed in phosphate buffer and subjected to the same extraction procedure).
[b] No difference was found between the alum-precipitated and the methylated bovine serum albumin—complexed forms (5).
[c] Some experiments were done with mouse and guinea pig PE cells.
[d] These experiments were done with PE cells from CBA and C57 mice.
[e] 1 part of radioactive compound was diluted with 100 parts of cold hormone on a weight basis.

There was no correlation between RNA association and immunogenicity but rather between binding and the charge of the antigen. All the molecules bearing negative charges (poly-glutamic acid, IgG, carboxylated dextran, poly (tyr, glu)-poly-DL-ala—polylys (TGAL), glutamic acid) showed some association in contrast to uncharged molecules (dextran, testosterone, estradiol and cortisone) regardless of their size, complexity and immunogenicity. The RNA could not be saturated by increasing the antigen-RNA ratio within practical limits, suggesting that the RNA involved was not specific. Moreover, the synthetic polypeptide (TGAL) was binding to the same extent to P. E. cells RNA from mice of strain C57 which are good responders to this polypeptide and from strain CBA which are poor responders [10, 12].

Kinetics of Association between Antigen and RNA

Using the same number of P. E. cells from the same rabbit in order to minimize trivial differences, the kinetics of antigen-RNA association were studied by varying the incubation time from 1 min to 48 hours and the temperature from 2° C to 37° C. No significant differences were found in antigen-RNA ratios or the efficiencies of binding under those conditions. The same findings were also obtained whether cell homogenates were used instead of living cells and when these homogenates were subjected to treatment with pronase or dithiothreitol or to a temperature of 80° C for 5 min or when they were incubated with antigen in the presence of 0.5% sodium dodecyl sulfate.

These results [10] suggested that the formation of RNA-antigen complexes was not an enzyme-mediated reaction and hence rendered unlikely covalent binding between RNA and antigen.

Association and RNA Synthesis

In experiments in which nuclei and mitochondria were removed from P. E. cell homogenates and the remaining fraction incubated with antigen, the efficiency of binding was the same as when unfractionated homogenates were used.

When transcription was blocked by actinomycin D, as shown by the lack of ^{14}C-uridine incorporation into RNA, again no impairment of binding was observed.

These results [10] confirmed that there is no need for RNA synthesis after the introduction of antigen to form complexes, as had already been reported earlier [4, 5, 13]. They also indicate that association of antigen to RNA is merely a passive phenomenon. The confirmation of this point and of the non-covalent nature of the bond was provided using purified RNA. An association, qualitatively and quantitatively identical to that found *in vivo*, could take place *in vitro* provided that Mg^{++} ions were present [10]. The characteristics of association and dissociation between purified RNA and negatively charged molecules suggested that the binding was due to chelation of divalent cations by anionic groups on the RNA and "antigen" moiety of the complexes.

Formation of Antigen Complexes with RNA from P. E., HeLa and E. coli Cells

In another series of experiments the significance of the lower density band of ribonucleoprotein found by zonal sedimentation in cesium sulfate was investigated. The synthetic polypeptide TGAL was incubated with homogenates of rabbit, guinea pig, C57 and CBA mice P. E., HeLa or E. coli cells. The RNA was extracted with cold phenol [9] or hot phenol [14] and submitted to zonal sedimentation in cesium sulfate [9].

In all gradients a major band of RNA was observed at a density of 1.68. After hot phenol treatment this was the only band seen in the gradient. After cold phenol extraction one or two "minor bands" were found at densities ranging from 1.56 to 1.63. In contrast Gottlieb described a minor band with a constant density of 1.588

whether using T2 phage or a synthetic copolymer glu-ala-tyr or no antigen at all, although quite surprisingly, in the same gradients the density of pure RNA ("major band") varied between 1.620 and 1.676 [5, 6, 7, 8].

When ^{125}I-labelled TGAL was used, radiolabel was associated with the RNA extracted by cold phenol and in cesium sulfate appeared concentrated in the "minor band" and free at the top of the gradient. When hot phenol was used no radiolabel was detected in the RNA preparation. When no antigen was used the lower density band was also present after the cold phenol extraction but absent when hot phenol was used. The important point was that the same amount of ^{125}I-TGAL was bound by RNA from P.E., HeLa or E. coli cells and in each case the complexes appeared as a minor band of lower density in cesium sulfate. The immunogenicity or adjuvant-icity of the RNA bands isolated from several cell species are under investigation. Preliminary results seem to show that the E. coli RNA is more active than that of P.E. or HeLa cells. These findings clearly show that the formation of antigen-RNA preparation depends on the method used for RNA preparation and is not specific for macrophages. Moreover, protein-RNA appears as a minor band also in the absence of antigen.

A Physiologically Significant Role for Macrophage RNA-Antigen Complexes in Immune Induction?

Several facets of antigen-RNA association have been examined: the formation of complexes was unrelated to the immunopotency of the antigen, was not an enzyme dependent reaction, did not involve covalent binding, did not require RNA synthesis following introduction of the antigen, did not involve antigen specific-RNA, but depended on the method used for RNA preparation and was not specific for macrophages.

Specificity was absent at every level examined: the antigen, the RNA, the association mechanism and the cell involved. This makes, in our opinion, an important physiological role for those complexes very unlikely. The association between antigen and RNA within viable cells has never been demonstrated and the RNA extraction procedure involves disrupting the organization of the cell: the most direct explanation for the appearance of these "antigen-RNA complexes" is that they represent artefacts of preparation.

There is strong immunochemical evidence against a major role in immune induction for small antigen fragments such as present on P.E. cells ribonucleoprotein complexes. (a) There is an inverse correlation between the electrical charge of the antigen and that of the antibody it elicits. In the case of antihapten antibody this correlation depends on the net overall charge of the antigen rather than the charge within the limited area around the haptenic determinant (reviewed in [15]). (b) Antigenic determinants are mostly conformation dependent (reviewed in [15] and [16]). (c) The response to a hapten is highly carrier specific [17] and requires the recognition of determinants on the carrier in addition to the haptenic determinant itself [18]. Thus the recognition of most antigenic determinants and the triggering of the immune response takes place while the immunogenic molecule is still intact and not after breakdown.

The enhanced potency of some antigens when complexed to RNA is not so surprising. It is well known that aggregating antigen or making it insoluble (e. g. by alum precipitation, by coating on bentonite, to give but two of a variety of methods) intensifies the antibody response. On the other hand the adjuvant action of polynucleotides seems to be also well established [19—21]. Of relevance to a hypothesis giving an essential specific role to macrophages in antigen recognition is the observation that macrophages from normal donors, after incubation with antigen, cannot elicit antibody production by lymphocytes from tolerant animals; yet macrophages from tolerant animals are fully effective in priming normal recipients (reviewed in [22]).

All this makes us look for another mechanism for macrophage-lymphocyte cooperation. Studies on the association of undegraded antigen with macrophage cell membrane and the increased immunogenicity of macrophage bound antigen may indicate that the role of the macrophage is not to process the antigen but to expose it in a more effective way to lymphoid cells [22—26]. Although this hypothesis is unable to account for all the observations [27] it has the advantages to be compatible with the immunochemical evidences on immune induction and that the experiments leading to it were performed under quasi physiological conditions.

Acknowledgements

I wish to thank Dr. B. A. ASKONAS for helpful discussion in the preparation of this manuscript.

References

1. FISHMAN, M.: J. exp. Med. 114, 837 (1961).
2. — ADLER, F. L.: J. exp. Med. 117, 595 (1963).
3. FRIEDMAN, H. P., STAVITSKY, A. B., SOLOMON, J. M.: Science 149, 1106 (1965).
4. ASKONAS, B. A., RHODES, J. M.: Nature 205, 470 (1965).
5. GOTTLIEB, A. A., GLISIN, V. R., DOTY, P.: Proc. nat. Acad. Sci. (Wash.) 57, 1849 (1967).
6. — R.E.S.J. Reticuloendothel. Soc. 5, 270 (1968).
7. — in: Nucleic Acid in Immunology. Eds.: O. J. PLESCIA and W. BRAUN. New York: Springer 1968, p. 471.
8. — Biochemistry 8, 2111 (1969).
9. ROELANTS, G. E., GOODMAN, J. W.: Biochemistry 7, 1432 (1968).
10. — — J. exp. Med. 130, 557 (1969).
11. — in: Biological Effects of Polynucleotides. Proceedings of the Fourth International Symposium on Molecular Biology. Eds.: R. F. BEERS und W. BRAUN. New York: Springer 1971 (in press).
12. McDEVITT, H. O., SELA, M.: J. exp. Med. 122, 517 (1965).
13. RASKA, K., COHEN, E. O.: Nature 217, 720 (1968).
14. SCHERRER, K., DARNELL, J. E.: Biochem. biophys. Res. Commun. 7, 486 (1962).
15. SELA, M.: Science 166, 1365 (1969).
16. GOODMAN, J. W.: Imunochemistry 6, 139 (1969).
17. MITCHISON, N. A., in: Cold Spring Harbor Symposium on Quantitative Biology 13, 431 (1967).
18. RAJEWSKY, K., SCHIRRMACHER, V., NASE, S., JERNE, N. K.: J. exp. Med. 129, 1131 (1969).
19. HILLEMAN, M. R., in: Biological Effects of Polynucleotides. Proceedings of the Fourth International Symposium on Molecular Biology. Eds.: R. F. BEERS and W. BRAUN. New York: Springer 1971 (in press).

20. Mozes, E., Shearer, G., in: Biological Effects of Polynucleotides. Proceedings of the Fourth International Symposium on Molecular Biology. Eds.: R. F. Beers and W. Braun. New York: Springer 1971 (in press).
21. Johnson, A. G., in: Biological Effects of Polynucleotides. Proceedings of the Fourth International Symposium on Molecular Biology. Eds.: R. F. Beers and W. Braun. New York: Springer 1971 (in press).
22. Askonas, B. A., Auzins, I., Unanue, E. R.: Bull. Soc. Chim. biol. (Paris) 50, 1113 (1968).
23. Unanue, E. R., Askonas, B. A.: J. exp. Med. 127, 915 (1968).
24. — — Immunology 15, 287 (1968).
25. — Cerottini, J.-C., Bedford, M.: Nature 222, 1193 (1969).
26. — — J. exp. Med. 131, 711 (1970).
27. Askonas, B. A., Jaroskova, L., in: Mononuclear Phagocytes. Ed.: van Furth. Blackwell 1970 (in press).

In vitro Studies of Cellular Co-Operation during Immune Induction

K.-U. HARTMANN

Introduction

The immune response, the activation of lymphoid cells by antigen, has been studied in various *in vitro* systems. For example, specific antigen stimulates lymphoid cells from sensitized animals to incorporate thymidine and to produce non-antibody substances (lymphokines) which will affect the behaviour of other cells (WOLSTENCROFT et al., this symposium). I shall discuss the ability of lymphoid cells to elaborate antibody *in vitro*, and describe the induction of haemolysin synthesis during the primary immune response of cultured mouse spleen cells to foreign erythrocytes.

Methodology

The basic experimental system has been described by MISHELL and DUTTON [1]. Spleen cell suspensions from normal, non-immunised mice are dispersed in enriched medium and kept in culture in the presence of immunogenic erythrocytes. 4 to 5 days later, the number of antibody-producing cells (PFC) is estimated by the direct local haemolysin assay [2]; this assay recognizes predominantly 19S or IgM-producing cells but none or only a few of the IgG-producing cells. The rise of the number of PFC during the first 4 to 5 days of the incubation seems to run parallel with similar events *in vivo* during the response of mouse spleens to the injection of erythrocytes: 500 to 2000 PFC are detected after 4 days of incubation of spleen cell suspensions with antigen. Different cells are present in the spleen cell suspensions, and it is likely that there is cellular cooperation in this immune response. I shall discuss the use of fractionated cell populations to study the possible role of cellular interactions during this *in vitro* response.

Separation of Attached and Non-Attached Cells

Incubation of the spleen cell suspension for 1 hour in Petri dishes at 37° C allows some of the cells (about 40%) to adhere to the plastic surface [3, 4]; the rest of the cells stay in suspension. The adhering subpopulation consists of endothelial cells, macrophages, and other cells; the non-adherent cells are predominantly small lymphocytes. Neither subpopulation alone gives a good response, as only a few PFC are detected after the 4-day incubation period (Table 1). However, combination of the two subpopulations allows the development of PFC.

Several experiments have been undertaken to analyze this situation. First, using subpopulations of different mouse strains which differ in histocompatibility antigens, it was shown that the PFC came from the non-adherent fraction: for the PFC carried the same H-antigens as did the non-adherent cells. Second, the adherent population could be irradiated with 1000 r without destruction of its ability to help the response. Third, the adherent cell population could be replaced by small numbers of peritoneal macrophages (Table 2) [4, 5] or even by the supernatant medium of attached cells. Thus it seems that the adhering cells are cooperating with the other cells in the response by adding some product which assists the reponse. It is not known if such products actually intiate or merely amplify the response: for they might act before induction, by changing the immunogenicity of the erythrocytes. On the other hand, they might increase the sensitivity of the precursor cells or assist proliferation of clones of antibody-producing cells.

Table 1

| | Non-attached cells | | | |
	—	0.8×10^6	1.6×10^6	5×10^6
—		—	0	0	120
Attached cells (2×10^6)	10	91	258	1400
Supernatant medium of attached cells		25	280	1570
	PFC/culture			

Table 2

Non-attached cells	Peritoneal exudate cells	PFC/10^6/day 5
4×10^6	—	54
4×10^6	2×10^4	53
4×10^6	6×10^4	326
4×10^6	1×10^5	2500
4×10^6	2×10^5	2170
4×10^6	8×10^5	90

Cell Fractionation Using Bovine Serum Albumin (BSA) Gradients

Fractionation of spleen cells was undertaken in BSA [6, 7] and Ficoll [8] gradients. Again it was shown that the precursor-rich cell fractions (D band fractions in the discontinuous BSA gradient) [6] could respond better in the presence of another cell fraction, the A-band fraction (Table 3). The A band cells were also able to function after irradiation.

Table 3. *Restoration of the ability to respond to antigen when A band and D band are recombined.* (From MISHELL, R. I., DUTTON, R. W., RAIDT, D. J.: Cellular Immunology)

		D band cells			
		0	1.7×10^6	5×10^6	15×10^6
—		—	1	34	275
A band cells	0.13×10^6	—	—	—	376
	0.4×10^6	—	—	—	1078
	1.2×10^6	—	516	344	950
	5×10^6	75	—	—	—

$$\text{PFC}/10^6$$

Cooperation between Bone Marrow-Derived and Thymus-Derived Lymphoid Cells

It is clear that lymphoid cells of bone marrow and thymic dependence cooperate in the immune response. Thymectomized irradiated mice, injected with bone marrow cells, responded poorly to a variety of immunogens; however, the response of these animals can be restored to normal by the injection of thymus cells or the presence of thymus grafts (LEUCHARS, this symposium).

In the present system, neither bone marrow nor thymus cells could be kept in culture in the desired concentrations for the necessary length of time to undertake full *in vitro* studies. Therefore the bone marrow cells were injected into thymectomized irradiated animals, whose spleens were then taken as a selective source of marrow-derived cells (here called B cells). It should be made clear that in these spleens there are lymphoid cell descendants of the injected bone marrow; but in addition, there are haemopoietic cells, endothelial cells, and other radiation-resistant cells.

Thymus cells were injected into irradiated mice together with foreign erythrocytes [9, 10], and 8 days later spleen cell suspensions were made from these animals (T cells). It was assumed that these spleen cell suspensions contained antigen sensitive cells that had been selected, activated or triggered by sequestered erythrocyte antigen. Only thymus-derived cells that had "seen" antigen in the host in this way were found to cooperate in the experimental system. These cells were called "educated" T cells.

Table 4 shows that very few PFC could be detected in cultures of B or T cells stimulated by SRBC; however, many PFC developed when cultures contained mixtures of B and T cells. These PFC were descendants of the B cell population, for they carried the corresponding histocompatibility markers: if the B cells were incubated with anti H-2 serum before the haemolysis assay, there was considerable reduction of PFC, due to inhibition of the B cells by the antiserum treatment (Table 5).

Furthermore, part of the response was dependent on the strain of origin of the T cells; addition of DBA T-cells promoted the development of more PFC from DBA and C57BL B-cells than did addition of C57BL T-cells.

Table 4. *Cooperation between sensitized thymus cells and bone marrow-derived spleen cells in vitro*

Spleen cell suspension (Exp. 247)		Immunogen (3×10^6 erythrocytes)	PFC/10^6 assayed with	
B cells	T cells		SRBC	HRBC
1.1×10^7	—	SRBC	7	0
1.1×10^7	—	HRBC	0	0
—	3.2×10^6 (I)	SRBC+HRBC	0	0
6×10^6	1.6×10^6 (I)	SRBC	420	4
6×10^6	1.6×10^6	HRBC	0	20
—	4×10^6 (II)	SRBC+HRBC	0	0
6×10^6	2×10^6 (II)	SRBC	20	0
6×10^6	2×10^6	HRBC	5	475

B cells: Mice thymectomized, irradiated (850 r) and injected with bone marrow cells 17 days before the experiment.

T cells: Mice irradiated (650 r) and injected with 5×10^7 thymus cells and 10^7 SRBC (group I) or 10^7 HRBC (group II) 7 days before the experiment.

Cells cultivated 4 days in the presence of the erythrocytes; PFC assay against SRBC and HRBC.

Table 5. *Anti H-2 sera analysis of the phenotype of PFC obtained in cultures of bone marrow-derived and thymus-derived spleen cells obtained from different strains of mice*

Cell suspension (Exp. 259)			PFC per culture (day 5) [a] assayed after treatment [b] with		
B cells	T cells		NMS	Anti H-2 b	Anti H-2 d
$C_{57}Bl$ (15×10^6)	—		45	0	30
—	$C_{57}Bl$	(8×10^6)	10	0	10
$C_{57}Bl$ (8×10^6)+	$C_{57}Bl$	(4×10^6)	110	0	145
$C_{57}Bl$ (8×10^6)+	DBA	(2×10^6)	515	75	380
DBA (9×10^6)	—		40	30	0
—	DBA	(4×10^6)	20	30	0
DBA (5×10^6)+	DBA	(2×10^6)	840	700	10
DBA (5×10^6)+	$C_{57}Bl$	(4×10^6)	260	210	20
Normal spleen cells:					
$C_{57}Bl/6$ spleen (17×10^6)			800	105 (13%)	900
DBA/2 spleen (15×10^6)			2500	2500	230 (9%)

B cells: Mice thymectomized, irradiated with 850 r, injected with 3×10^7 isogeneous bone marrow cells.

T cells: Mice irradiated with 750 r and injected with 5×10^7 thymus cells and SRBC.

[a] At the beginning of the culture period 3×10^6 SRBC were added.

[b] The cells were harvested, centrifuged and resuspended in the original volume. 0.2 ml cell suspension was incubated with 25 µl normal mouse serum (NMS) or anti H-2 sera, 30 min at 0°. After washing in 5 ml BSS addition of 25 µl guinea pig serum, incubation 15 min at 35° C. After washing in 5 ml ice cold BSS assay of the PFC.

Cooperation was possible only if the erythrocytes which were used to educate the T cells were also present in the cultures. Table 6 shows that there was non-specific spread of the stimulatory effects of educated T cells. In this experiment, SRBC-educated and horse (HRBC)-educated T cells were mixed with the B cells, singly, and in combination. In the presence of both kinds of erythrocytes, the T cells were able to assist the development of PFC against both erythrocytes. There was no cross reaction between the two kinds of erythrocytes; in fact, SRBC-educated T cells did not help anti HRBC response alone, and *vice versa* (Table 6).

Table 6

B cells	T cells	Immunogen	PFC/10^6/day 4 against	
			SRBC (sheep)	HRBC (horse)
10×10^6	—	SRBC+HRBC	22	8
—	7.0×10^6	SRBC+HRBC	49	0
5.0×10^6	3.5×10^6	SRBC	450	21
5.0×10^6	3.5×10^6	HRBC	14	29
5.0×10^6	3.5×10^6	SRBC+HRBC	1010	250

T cells: F_1 mice, irradiated (600 r), injected with 5×10^7 thymus cells and 10^7 SRBC 9 days before the experiment (# 242).
SRBC: Sheep erythrocytes. — HRBC: Horse erythrocytes.

Discussion

It was particularly interesting that the SRBC-educated T cells, in the presence of SRBC, were able to cooperate with B cells to allow the development of SRBC-PFC and also the development of HRBC-PFC. It is thought that the precursor cells are already determined to recognize SRBC or HRBC as antigen; thus, it seems that the stimulated T cells (SRBC-educated T cells incubated together with SRBC) are able to help the induction or clone formation from sensitized B cells (i. e., sensitized by SRBC or HRBC). It is not known what these T cells add to the system, but it is possible that they are releasing some factors, which either act directly on the precursor cells (e. g. nutritional or mitogenic factors) or indirectly on other cells (e. g. macrophages). It is tempting to speculate that the active factors are lymphokines (Wolstencroft et al., this symposium) which are released by the stimulated T cells, and that it is these factors which explain part of the stimulatory activity.

These present results are also compatible with other findings. Firstly, spleen cells of newborn-thymectomized mice give a low response to SRBC; but the response could be restored by addition of irradiated non-attached cells [11]. Secondly, thymus cells are necessary to restore the response in spleen cells of bone marrow chimeras [12]. Thirdly, this response could be suppressed by anti-theta serum [13], presumably acting by inhibiting the thymus-derived cell population.

The methods utilized in this study have allowed enrichment or depletion of precursor cells in spleen cell populations. With erythrocytes as immunogen, it is clear that optimal *in vitro* development of PFC from the precursor-enriched sub-population needed the help of other cells. Little is known about the function of these helping cells: it is not known whether they act preferentially during the inductive or the proliferative phase of the response. It seems likely that soluble substances released from the attached cell population, even in the absence of antigen, and that factors derived from antigen-stimulated thymus-derived cells, may both be involved in the cooperative phenomena. It is hoped that further extension of cell fractionation techniques and modifications to the design of these *in vitro* systems will yield more decisive information about the molecular and cellular basis for regulation of the antibody response.

Acknowledgements

The skilful technical assistance and cooperation of Mrs S. Regg, Miss C. Mehner and Mrs E. Zappe is gratefully acknowledged. This work was supported in part by the Deutsche Forschungsgemeinschaft, grant Ha 569/3.

References

1. Mishell, R. I., Dutton, R. W.: J. exp. Med. 126, 423 (1967).
2. Jerne, N. K., Nordin, A. A., Henry, C., in: Cell bound antibodies. Eds.: B. Amos and H. Koprowski. Philadelphia 1963, p. 109.
3. Mosier, D. E.: Science 158, 1575 (1967).
4. Hartman, K.-U., Dutton, R. W., McCarthy, Margareth, M., Mishell, R. I.: Cellular Immunology, in press.
5. Hoffmann, M.: Immunology 18, 791 (1970).
6. Mishell, R. I., Dutton, R. W., Raidt, D. J.: Cellular Immunology, in press.
7. Hashill, J. S.: J. exp. Med. 130, 877 (1969).
8. Schimpl, A., Wecker, E.: Personal comm.
9. Clamann, H. N., Chaperon, E. A., Triplett, R. F.: Proc. Soc. exp. Biol. (N.Y.) 122, 167 (1966).
10. Miller. J. F. A. P., Mitchell, G. F.: J. exp. Med. 128, 801 (1968).
11. Hirst, J. A., Dutton, R. W.: Cellular Immunology, in press.
12. Munro, A., Hunter. P.: Nature 255, 277 (1970).
13. Schimpl, A., Wecker, E.: Nature 226, 1258 (1970).

Lymphocyte Mitogenic Factor in Cell-Mediated Immunity

R. A. Wolstencroft, M. Matthew, C. Oates, R. N. Maini, and D. C. Dumonde

With 2 Figures

Introduction

One of the most striking recent advances in immunobiology is the recognition that immune induction is regulated by cellular interactions between physiologically distinct compartments of the lymphoid system (for refs. see [3, 4, 15]); and the mechanisms involved provide for interactions between macrophages and lymphocytes, and between thymus-dependent lymphocytes and other lymphocytes, in the antibody-producing response of the lymphoid system to antigen. Recent analysis of cell-mediated immune reactions strongly suggests that cellular interactions also play an important part in their mechanism (for refs. see [7]). The concept of cellular co-operation is fundamental to the organisation of anything but the simplest of multi-cellular organisms [19]; and, in biological terms, the organisation of the cell-mediated immune response can be no exception. The recent concept which gives rise to this discussion relates to evidence that cellular co-operation in cell-mediated immunity may in fact be regulated by non-antibody mediators generated during the process of lymphocyte activation [7, 11]. During the last few years, experimental methods have been developed for the recognition and assay of such biologically active factors; and in this paper we shall discuss the induction, nature and specificity of one of these biological activities, which we have termed "lymphocyte mitogenic factor". As might be anticipated, the recognition of this factor emerged from studies on the possible role of a soluble mediator in the phenomenon of antigen directed lymphocyte transformation [6, 21, 22]. In this paper we shall describe the generation of lymphocyte mitogenic factor in three widely different animal species; laboratory rodents, chickens, and Man.

Methodology

The general procedure involves obtaining lymphocyte suspensions from putatively sensitized animals or Man and culturing them together with antigens to which the animal or human subject is thought to have developed cell-mediated immunity. Some time before the peak of the lymphocyte transformation response, which varies for different species, the lymphocytes are centrifuged from the culture, and the supernatants are harvested. The supernatants are then tested for their ability to activate the DNA metabolism of fresh populations of lymphocytes obtained from unsensitized members of the homologous species. As a necessary biological control, a second aliquot of the original donor lymphocyte population is cultured in the same way, but without the addition of antigen to the cell suspension. After removing the lymphocytes, specific antigen is now added to this control culture supernatant to "reconstitute" it to the same concentration of antigen that was present in the other ("preincubated") supernatant. The experiments by which lymphocyte mitogenic factor is recognized consist in determining whether the DNA metabolism of the fresh lymphocytes is more active in the presence of the preincubated lymphocyte supernatant than in the presence of its corresponding reconstituted control. In practice, it is convenient to measure lymphocyte activation by incorporation of tritiated thymidine over an 18-hour period preceding the termination of the "test" cultures; and to employ various dilutions of the preincubated and reconstituted lymphocyte supernatants, in tissue culture medium, to reveal the strength of the lymphocyte mitogenic factor. The activity of the mitogenic factor is assessed by liquid scintillation counting of the incorporation of tritiated thymidine into the test lymphocytes, under defined conditions of isotope concentration and cell density. The results are evaluated in terms of the numerical difference between the incorporation rates induced by preincubated and reconstituted supernatants, measured as disintegrations per minute, or the numerical ratio of these values. The immunological specificity of the induction and expression of this lymphocyte mitogenic factor can therefore be evaluated by ringing the changes on the specificity of antigen: cell interaction, and on the immunological sensitivity of animals or Man providing the sources of "donor" and "recipient" lymphocytes.

Biochemical fractionation of the preincubated and reconstituted supernatants is done in parallel with each other and corresponding fractions are tested at equivalent dilutions in fresh tissue culture medium for their ability to stimulate incorporation of tritiated thymidine by fresh homologous lymphocytes, usually obtained from a non-sensitive subject. An important technical advance has been to induce lymphocyte mitogenic factor by culturing the donor lymphocytes in tissue culture media without the addition of serum supplements. By this procedure, the occurrence of the lymphocyte mitogenic factor in chromatographic or electrophoretic fractions is no longer swamped by the distribution of large amounts of added serum protein.

Lymphocyte Mitogenic Factor in the Guinea Pig (Table 1)

Lymphocyte cell suspensions are prepared from the draining lymph nodes of individual guinea pigs immunized two weeks earlier with protein antigen (e. g. bovine-gamma-globulin) in Freund's complete adjuvant. Preincubated and reconstituted supernatants are then prepared and assayed in corresponding dilution on fresh lymph node cells also obtained from guinea pigs immunized with similar or dissimilar antigens emulsified with adjuvants, or from guinea pigs injected with adjuvants alone. Mitogenic activity is demonstrable only when the donor lymphocytes are cultured with the antigen used for sensitization; however, its stimulating effect is equally apparent when tested on sensitive or non-sensitive recipient lymphocyte populations (Table 1).

In order to differentiate lymphocyte mitogenic factor from soluble transplantation antigens, we showed that mitogenic factor could stimulate an animal's own lymphocytes. Preincubated and reconstituted supernatants were prepared from the biopsied axillary and subscapular lymph nodes taken from single immunized animals. The inguinal and popliteal lymph nodes were taken on the following day and cultured in the presence of prepared supernatants. Here again, only when the supernatants were induced with the specific immunizing antigen was a mitogenic effect demonstrated (Table 1; [21]).

Table 1. *Specificity of induction and expression of guinea pig lymphocyte mitogenic factor.* (Data of Wolstencroft and Dumonde, 1970a)

Relation between sensitivity of "donor" and "recipient" lymphocytes	Corresponding specificity of antigen in culture supernatants	Lymphocyte mitogenic factor: Increased uptake (P-R) of ^{3}H-thymidine (d.p.m.) by recipient lymphocytes		
Similar	Donor and recipient	$+415\pm505$	(N=28;	P<0.001)
Dissimilar	Donor only	$+476\pm445$	(N=16;	P<0.001)
Dissimilar	Recipient only	-127 ± 351	(N=11;	P=0.3)
Similar or dissimilar	Unrelated antigen	$-\ 71\pm208$	(N=11;	P=0.3)
Identical (i. e. autologous)	Sensitizing antigen	$+460\pm402$	(N=\ 9;	P=0.01)
	Unrelated antigen	-245 ± 335	(N=\ 5;	P=0.2)

By this means it is possible to show the production of lymphocyte mitogenic factor by peripheral lymphocytes, lymph node cells, spleen cells and peritoneal exudate cells of sensitized guinea pigs. We have found it particularly convenient to assay the activity of this factor using lymph node cells; and these are simply derived from animals injected with saline emulsions of incomplete or complete Freund's adjuvants, to increase the yield of lymphocytes for the test procedure [22].

Lymphocyte Mitogenic Factor in the Chicken (Table 2)

In collaboration with Dr L. N. Payne, at the Houghton Poultry Research Station Huntingdon, chickens were sensitized with avian mycobacteria in oil, by intramuscular injection, at 7—12 weeks of age. Three weeks later, wattle tests with avian

Table 2. *Lymphocyte mitogenic factor in the chicken.* (Data of Oates et al., 1971)

Birds sensitized with avian tubercle	Mitogenic factor (Avian PPD)	Lymphocyte transformation	
		Avian PPD	PHA
Normal	7/7	7/7	7/7
Bursectomized (agammaglob.)	6/7	7/7	7/7
Thymectomized:			
Complete	1/4	0/4	1/4
Partial	4/4	1/4	2/4

tuberculin PPD showed that the birds had become tuberculin sensitive. At this time, heparinized blood was obtained by cardiac puncture and contaminating red cells were removed by repeated centrifugation of the buffy layer. The resulting leucocyte suspensions contained approximately 60% lymphocytes; and preincubated and reconstituted supernatants were generated with avian PPD (Weybridge) in 3-day cultures. The supernatants were tested for lymphocyte mitogenic factor using fresh peripheral blood lymphocytes from unsensitized chickens [16].

The importance of using the chicken lies in the ability to undertake studies of bursectomy and thymectomy. These surgical operations were carried out by Dr L. N. PAYNE in one-day-old chicks and the birds were irradiated with 900 r one day later. When the birds had reached 7 weeks of age, they were sensitized with avian mycobacteria in oil by intramuscular injection and their peripheral blood lymphocytes were tested for the production of mitogenic factor 3 weeks after sensitization, by culture with standard amounts of avian PPD. The preincubated and reconstituted supernatants made in this way were tested on allogeneic lymphocytes from unsensitized normal birds. The bursectomized birds were agammaglobulinaemic and gave no primary or secondary antibody responses to sheep erythrocytes; but their lymphocytes were just as active in producing lymphocyte mitogenic factor as cells from normal tuberculin sensitive birds (Table 2). Complete surgical thymectomy is technically difficult; and histological examination of thymectomized birds on a later occasion showed that some had thymic remnants which survived operation. The effect of complete thymectomy was to suppress the production of mitogenic factor and lymphocyte transformation to PPD; and partial thymectomy was more successful at suppressing the complete lymphocyte transformation than suppressing the production of mitogenic factor which could be revealed by its ability to activate normal lymphocytes (Table 2). These studies in the chicken therefore show that the production of lymphocyte mitogenic factor by antigen stimulation is independent of that compartment of the lymphoid system which is concerned with antibody production; and the results of these investigations support the concept that lymphocyte mitogenic factor is part of the lymphokine group of non-antibody mediators of cellular immunity [7]. Further preliminary studies have shown that the peripheral blood lymphocytes of sensitized bursectomized birds are capable of generating migration inhibition factor, active on spleen explants from normal birds, when the lymphocytes are cultured with sensitizing antigen (avian tuberculin). In fact, this latter observation takes one stage further the interesting work of ARONSON (1931) who showed that the migration of cells from bone marrow explants of tuberculous birds could be inhibited by the addition of tuberculin to the culture medium.

Lymphocyte Mitogenic Factor in Man (Table 3)

The production of soluble mitogenic factor during antigen activation of human peripheral blood lymphocytes was shown by the culture of lymphocytes with tuberculin PPD from donors with known clinical hypersensitivity to the antigen [12]. By assaying preincubated and reconstituted supernatants in parallel, we showed that when the lymphocyte donor was known to be positive, the mitogenic factor had the property of stimulating DNA synthesis of allogeneic lymphocytes

Table 3. *Lymphocyte mitogenic factor in tuberculin sensitive and grass-pollen allergic subjects.* (Data of Maini et al., 1969, 1970)

Antigen induction	Mantoux:		Grass-pollen	
	Positive	Negative	Allergic	Non-allergic
Lymphocyte transformation:				
PPD	28/30	1/16		
Grass pollen antigen			22/24	2/18
Mitogenic factor:				
PPD	20/23	2/19		
Grass pollen antigen			21/24	4/18

derived from Mantoux-negative or other Mantoux-positive donors. Moreover, mitogenic factor activity could be demonstrated on autologous lymphocytes on a subsequent occasion; the stimulation of DNA synthesis was greater than that which could be accounted for by the amount of antigen present in the reconstituted control culture supernatant. Autologous testing for mitogenic factor in Man is likely to be the best method for its demonstration as it overcomes the possible involvement of solubilized transplantation antigens which could independently stimulate DNA synthesis of allogeneic human lymphocytes [9]. The elaboration of mitogenic factor can easily be seen after 3 days of lymphocyte culture with antigen; and this is followed at 5—6 days by a peak of blast cell transformation of the lymphocyte population. It is of interest that antigen-induced lymphocyte transformation occurs not only when a delayed type of skin sensitivity is present (e. g. tuberculin) but also when immediate hypersensitivity is the only observable skin response [8]. We have found that mitogenic factor is generated in culture supernatants of lymphocytes derived from subjects with grass pollen allergy, upon culture with mixed grass pollen antigens [13]. These grass pollen sensitive subjects produce only an immediate hypersensitivity reaction at the site of allergen testing.

The demonstration of mitogenic factor production is conveniently undertaken by using column purified suspensions of human lymphocytes in which the proportion of erythrocytes to lymphocytes is about 2 : 1, and in which lymphocytes represent about 98—99% of the white cell populations. The demonstration that mitogenic factor production runs parallel with antigen-induced lymphocyte transformation in both delayed and immediate hypersensitivity suggests the possibility that there is more than one class of soluble mitogenic factor in Man.

Generation of Mitogenic Inhibitors in Culture

Products of simple lymphocyte culture contain materials which, if added to tissue culture medium containing fresh lymphocytes, frequently depress DNA metabolism, as judged by the incorporation of tritiated thymidine. We have found that in high concentration, both preincubated and reconstituted lymphocyte supernatants may actually depress thymidine incorporation by fresh lymphocytes; this feature can be true of lymphocytes obtained from rodents, chickens or Man. Part of this inhibitory activity may be due to nutritional depletion; and this is suggested by experiments in which inhibitory activity can be removed after 24 hours of dialysis (Fig. 1). The possibility that lymphocyte transformation is accompanied by the generation of soluble mediators which can both activate and limit the cellular response may be of importance in the regulation of cell-mediated immunity; however, it has yet to be determined whether these features are artifacts of culture procedures or whether cultured lymphocytes can generate a true mitotic inhibitor analogous to growth regulatory substances ("chalones") which appear to function in other biological systems [18].

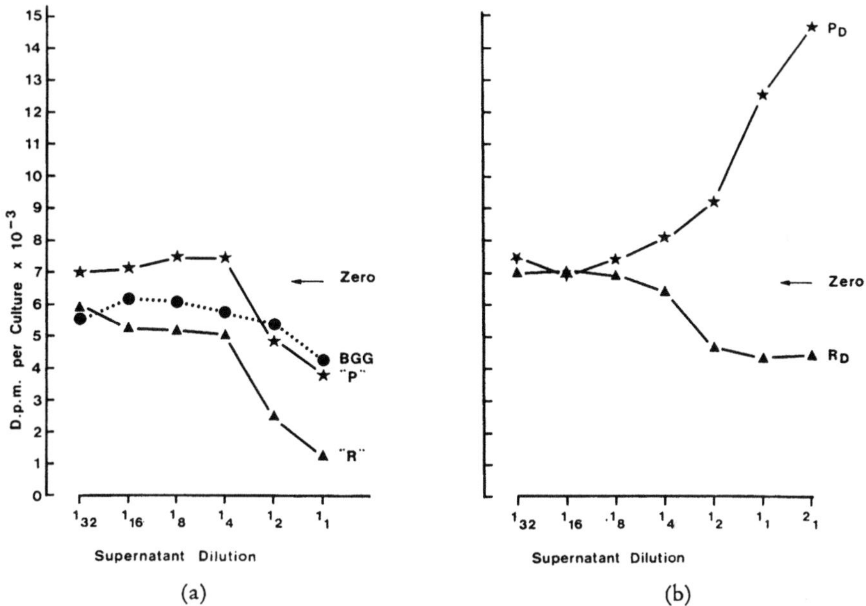

Fig. 1 a and b. Removal by dialysis of inhibitors of mitogenic factor from lymphocyte culture fluids. (a) "P" and "R": Preincubated and reconstituted supernatants before dialysis. BGG: Bovine γ-globulin antigen (1 mg/ml at 1/1 dilution). (b) "P$_D$" and "R$_D$": Preincubated and reconstituted supernatants after 24-hour dialysis. "Zero": Represents basal level of 3-H-thymidine incorporation of test lymphocytes

Biochemical Studies of Lymphocyte Mitogenic Factor

Recent improvements in culture methodology have permitted greater purification and characterization of mitogenic factor in the guinea pig. Firstly, serum has been eliminated from the donor cell cultures generating biological activity; second, oil-induced peritoneal exudate cells have been used in preference to lymph node cells because the amount of mitogenic activity generated is comparable and yet the un-dialysed supernatants at high concentration showed much less inhibition of thymidine incorporation by the test lymphocytes. Third, the inducing antigen (bovine γ-

globulin) is purified before being used in culture; a fraction of bovine γ-globulin is used that is precipitated by ammonium sulphate at 33% saturation, and is excluded from column chromatography on DEAE cellulose at 0.01 molar phosphate pH 7.9 [14].

Active supernatants prepared in this way were fractionated by stepwise ammonium sulphate precipitation at 0—40, 40—50, 50—80 and 80—100% saturation. The resulting precipitates were exhaustively dialysed free of salt, lyophilized, and finally reconstituted with tissue culture medium at concentrations comparable to the original supernatant volume. When tested on fresh recipient lymph node cells, the majority of the activity was localized in the 50—80% fraction; and by comparison with the weight of recovered material this fraction was shown to have a greatly increased specific activity. This simple fractionation procedure yields a 20-fold purification by comparison with the original supernatants and reveals lymphocyte mitogenic factor to be active down to a concentration of 1 µg/ml. Studies of ion exchange chromatography have revealed that mitogenic activity elutes from DEAE cellulose between 0.12-M and 0.4-M phosphate buffer pH 7.9, which provides an alternative procedure to separate it from the inducing antigen. Loss of total mitogenic activity sometimes occurs during purification procedures; thus we find a 23% loss of activity on fractional precipitation with ammonium sulphate. We consider this to be a feature of physiochemical denaturation as we have not been able to potentiate the activity of the 50—80% ammonium sulphate fraction either by recombination with the other fractions or by addition of an inducing antigen.

In culture supernatants containing serum, the mitogenic factor behaves with a molecular weight of 30—80,000 (by gel filtration) and runs with albumin and α_1-globulin on preparative acrylamide electrophoresis. Culture supernatants derived from tuberculin activated human lymphocytes contain mitogenic factor which distributes itself in a similar way on gel filtration and ammonium sulphate fractionation. As judged by parallel experiments with isotope-labelled antigens, it appears that lymphocyte mitogenic factor can be separated from nearly all antigen; and this feature, together with its physiochemical properties, reveal that it is quite distinct from classical immunoglobulin.

The biochemical relationship of lymphocyte mitogenic factor to other non-antibody lymphokine mediators of cellular immunity is of great interest [20]. Our purification studies of migration inhibition factor generated by guinea pig lymphocytes reveal certain physiochemical similarities between the distribution of these two activities. However, it has yet to be determined whether any one biological activity can be carried on different macromolecules; or whether a given macromolecule, generated by lymphocyte activation, can have multiple activities. We have freed migration-inhibition factor of antigen and contaminating serum protein by sequential immune precipitation; and we are now proceeding to apply this technique to the purification of lymphocyte mitogenic factor.

Immunological and Biological Significance of Lymphocyte Mitogenic Factor

Present evidence suggests that there are a group of soluble factors, generated by antigen activation of sensitized lymphocytes, which have activities relevant to the expression of cellular immunity and which are specifically induced but non-specifically expressed. These soluble factors are active after the removal of the sensitized cell population which generated them, without prejudice to the possibility that *in vivo* there may be a synergistic action between the soluble factors and original or succeeding populations of lymphoid cells. Biochemical evidence reveals that this class of cell-free activities is not dependent upon persistence of antigen or presence of classical immune complexes; and this is important, because the products of combination of antigen with classical antibody can also cause physiological and immunological activation of lymphoid cells [5]. We have given the term "lymphokine" to describe this wide range of biological activities which are generated under circumstances that also result in lymphocyte activation. In collaboration with Dr R. H. KELLY and Dr B. BALFOUR, of the National Institute for Medical Research, 100 µg quantities of guinea pig lymphokine factors were injected directly into the lymphatics of the guinea pig ear. Twenty-four hours later there was an 80% increase in lymph node weight and a 70% increase in cells expressable from preauricular draining lymph nodes [10]; and the histology of these lymph nodes showed great paracortical distension with squashing of germinal centres and the development of lymphocyte plugging in the cortico-medullary sinuses at this time. Under these circumstances, the soluble factors display effects on cellular traffic within the lymph node; and the nature of these cellular responses therefore provides a morphological justification for use of the generic term "lymphokine".

The demonstration that lymphokine factors act on lymphocytes, macrophages, fibroblasts, vascular endothelium and tissue cells clearly provides a basis for their participation in the peripheral expression of cell-mediated immunity [7]. Their rapidity of action and their biological effects suggest that the factors, including lymphocyte mitogenic factor, may initially act on cell membranes by modifying associations of macromolecules or enzyme systems in cell surfaces and thereby resulting in behavioural and metabolic changes in responding cells. The features of these changes will depend on the composition of cell populations and the local concentration of active mediators; and on this basis it may be possible to view the significance of lympokine factors as of fundamental importance in mechanisms of cellular surveillance [2].

At a more speculative basis, the generation of lymphocyte mitogenic factor and other mediators within lymphoid tissue may be expected to affect the immunological response. The possibility arises that the action of lymphocyte mitogenic factor may be of fundamental importance in maintaining antigen-sensitive cells of both lymphocyte compartments in a physiologically sensitive state; and by this means to facilitate co-operation between thymus-dependent lymphocytes and cells of direct bone marrow lineage (Fig. 2). Such a mechanism operating during the cellular response to antigen may be expected to lead to local activation of immunocytes of different antigenic specificities (see HARTMANN, this symposium p. 22); and it is tempting to ascribe to this mechanism some features of antibody heterogeneity, and even the production of non-specific immunoglobulin. On the other hand, over-production of soluble mediators might be expected to lead to desensitization of cell-mediated immunity or even to high-dose tolerence for the whole immune response, by some form of sterile activation analogous to the action of anti-lymphocyte serum. On this basis, the discovery of the lymphocyte activating (mitogenic) factor may have provided an important clue as to the biological significance of cellular immune mediators. It may be that the development of a humoral mechanism for mitotic activation of mobile cells constituted an important step in the evolution of the adaptive immune response; and that if such a lymphocyte mediator were found to act on metabolic DNA [17] this might yield a molecular basis for maintenance of immune flexibility despite the tendency for phenotypic restriction during the immune response.

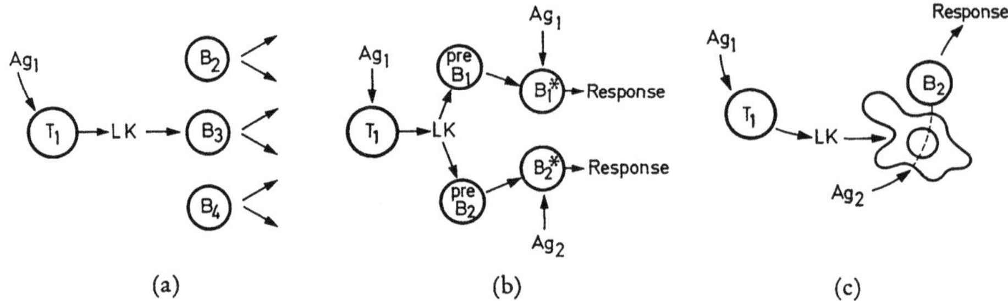

Fig. 2 a—c. Representations of possible role of lymphokine factors in cooperation between thymus dependent cells (T cells) and other lymphocytes (B cells). (a) and (b) suggest direct lymphocyte cooperation. (c) suggests additional participation of the macrophage. (See also HARTMANN; this symposium)

In conclusion, whether we prefer to view the lymphocyte mitogenic factor as a cell co-operator or as a traffic regulator, it is clearly involved in the peripheral expression of cell-mediated immunity. At present, we can only speculate as to its role in regulation of the immunological response and its significance in mechanisms of cellular surveillance. We would like to suggest that its phylogenetic development constituted an important step in the evolution of the adaptive immune response and to predict that the origin of the lymphokine system as a whole may run parallel with the development of adaptive immunity.

Acknowledgements

The work described in this paper is supported by grants from the Medical Research Council, the Arthritis and Rheumatism Council, and the Wellcome Foundation.

References

1. ARONSON, J. D.: J. exp. Med. 54, 387 (1931).
2. BURNET, F. M.: Cellular Immunology. Cambridge University Press 1969.
3. CLAMAN, H. N., CHAPERON, B. A., TRIPLETT, R. F.: Proc. Soc. exp. Biol. (N.Y.) 121, 236 (1966).
4. DAVIES, A. J. S.:Transplant. Rev. 1, 43 (1969).
5. DUMONDE, D. C.: Proc. roy. Soc. Med. 63, 934 (1970).
6. — HOWSON, W. T., WOLSTENCROFT, R. A.: 5th International Symposium on Immunopathology, 1967. Eds.: P. A. MIESCHER and P. GRABAR. Basel: Schwabe 1968, p. 263.
7. — WOLSTENCROFT, R. A., PANAYI, G. S., MATTHEW, M., MORLEY, J., HOWSON, W. T.: Nature 224, 38 (1969).
8. GIRARD, J. P., ROSE, N. R., KUNZ, M. L., KUBAYASHI, S., ARBESMAN, C. E.: J. Allergy 39, 65 (1967).
9. KASAKURA, T., LOWENSTEIN, L.: Nature 219, 652 (1968).

10. KELLY, R. H., BALFOUR, B., MATTHEW, M., DUMONDE, D. C.: To be published (1971).
11. LAWRENCE, H. S., LANDY, M., (eds.): Mediators of cellular immunity. New York: Academic Press 1969.
12. MAINI, R. N., BRYCESON, A. D. M., WOLSTENCROFT, R. A., DUMONDE, D. C.: Nature 224, 42 (1969).
13. — HARGREAVE, F. E., FAUX, J., PEPYS, J., DUMONDE, D. C.: Clin. exp. Immunol. (1971) in press.
14. MATTHEW, M., WOLSTENCROFT, R. A., PANAYI, G. S., PAGE, D. A., DUMONDE, D. C.: To be published (1971). See WOLSTENCROFT and DUMONDE, 1970a.
15. NOSSAL. G. J. V., CUNNINGHAM, A., MITCHELL, G. F., MILLER, J. F. A. P.: J. exp. Med. 128, 839 (1968).
16. OATES, C. M., MAINI, R. N., PAYNE, L. N., DUMONDE, D. C.: To be published (1971).
17. PELC, S. R.: J. cell. Sci. 3, 263 (1968).
18. TEIR, H., RYTÖMAA, T., (eds.): Control of cellular growth in adult organisms. London: Academic Press 1967.
19. WILLMER, E. N.: Cytology and evolution. New York: Academic Press 1960.
20. WOLSTENCROFT, R. A.: Proc. symp. organ transplantation, Lyon 1970. Ed.: J.-P. REVEILLARD. Basel: Karger 1970 (in press).
21. — DUMONDE, D. C.: Immunology 18, 599 (1970a).
22. — Proc. N. I. H. Workshop on methods in cell-mediated immunity, New York 1970. Ed.: B. BLOOM. In press (1970b).

The Uptake of Antigens and Non-Antigenic Markers by Mouse Spleen and Peritoneal Cells*

T. MANDEL and P. BYRT

With 3 Figures

The initial events in the induction of an immune response are poorly understood but it is generally believed that a response is initiated when antigens react with receptors located on the surface of lymphoid cells. It is also believed that these receptors are immunoglobulin molecules and recent work suggests that they may be IgM molecules [1]. However the precise location and distribution of these receptor sites is not clear.

Recently an attempt was made by NAOR and SULITZEANU to identify the cells binding antigen *in vitro*, by incubating spleen cells from unimmunized mice with radio iodinated bovine serum albumin and detecting the labelled cells by autoradiography [2]. They showed that about 1 nucleated cell in every 1500 was heavily labelled; the labelled cells were of quite variable morphology and included some typical lymphocytes.

BYRD and ADA [3] investigated various parameters of this reaction and examined cells from various lymphoid organs in the rat and the mouse. They confirmed that lymphoid cells were indeed labelled but noted that the numbers labelled varied widely depending on the source of the cells and on the dose and type of antigen used. In particular, they showed that in the mouse surprisingly high numbers of peritoneal "lymphocyte like" cells bound the antigen haemocyanin (*Jasus lalandii*) even under conditions when phagocytosis was inhibited. Furthermore this binding could be markedly reduced by prior exposure of the cells to a polyvalent anti mouse immunoglobulin. These data suggested that the antigen was indeed bound to the surface of lymphoid cells. They also demonstrated that at least a proportion of such labelled cells were biologically active since they could be specifically inactivated by self-irradiation by the bound radio iodinated antigen [4].

However, some aspects of the *in vitro* antigen binding reaction could not be elucidated by light microscopy because of the limited resolving power of the optical microscope. It was therefore decided to investigate this reaction using the greater resolving power of the electron microscope in order firstly to gain more information about the morphology of the cells binding antigen and secondly to locate more precisely the site and distribution of the antigen receptor areas. In addition it was possible to use mixtures of markers, both immunogens and non-immunogens in order

---

* This is Publication No. 1449 from the Walter & Eliza Hall Institute.

to determine whether the cells showed any degree of selectivity for the various particles to which they were exposed. Some preliminary ultra structural data have been reported elsewhere [5].

The cells used in this study were obtained from the spleens and unstimulated peritoneal cavity of unprimed young adult (C57 Bl×CBA) hybrid mice. Cell suspensions were exposed to various mixtures of the markers for periods ranging from 10 min to 4 hours but most commonly for 30 min. The cells were exposed in Eagles medium usually at 37° C and in the absence of any metabolic inhibitors in order to allow phagocytic cells full opportunity to ingest the markers. The markers used were the immunogens, flagellar protein from *Salmonella adelaide* and haemocyanin from *Jasus lalandii;* both of these were labelled with ^{125}I and were detected by electron microscope autoradiography, and the antigen horse spleen ferritin which could be seen directly in the electron microscope because of its electron dense iron core. The non-immunogenic particles used were colloidal gold chloride and, less commonly, colloidal carbon. Both these materials have an inherent electron density. Mixtures of particles were usually composed on an iodinated antigen, ferritin and colloidal gold.

After exposure of the cells to the markers, the cells were passed through a series of foetal calf serum gradients in order to remove unbound material. The cells were then gently centrifuged to form a loose pellet which was fixed in glutaraldehyde, post fixed in osmium and embedded in araldite. Ultra thin sections were cut and either processed for autoradiography using Kodak NTE emulsion or mounted on grids and examined directly in a Philips EM 300 electron microscope. Autoradiographs were exposed for suitable periods, developed in Dektol and examined unstained.

In the spleen cell suspensions a variety of intact nucleated cells, red blood cells and cell debris was seen.

Cell debris, either isolated pieces of cytoplasm, bare nuclei or obviously damaged cells were commonly labelled. Such damaged cells and debris appeared to be freely permeable to all the markers to which they were exposed and mixtures of the various particles were seen scattered diffusely. When markers were present at the surface of damaged cells they were usually uniformly distributed and showed no aggregation at particular sites. Bare nuclei were usually heavily labelled throughout their substance.

Of the intact cells very few were labelled. No red cells were seen which bound any marker and granulocytes were only occasionally lightly labelled. Lymphocytes, both medium and small, were common but the great majority showed no evidence of labelling. However, occasional morphologically typical small and medium lymphocytes were labelled with the immunogens but not with the non-immunogenic marker colloidal gold chloride. Typically such labelled lymphocytes were only labelled with one immunogen per cell and doubly labelled lymphocytes were not seen. The label on these cells was present at the cell surface and was invariably seen as a number of discrete isolated patches (Fig. 1). The number of patches per cell profile was variable and ranged from one or two up to 20 or more. However no cell was seen which appeared to be evenly coated with antigen. Autoradiography could not establish the precise localization of the antigen since a scatter of grains occurred straddling the cell surface. When ferritin was used greater resolution could be obtained and the antigen molecules were seen just outside the visible limit of the cell

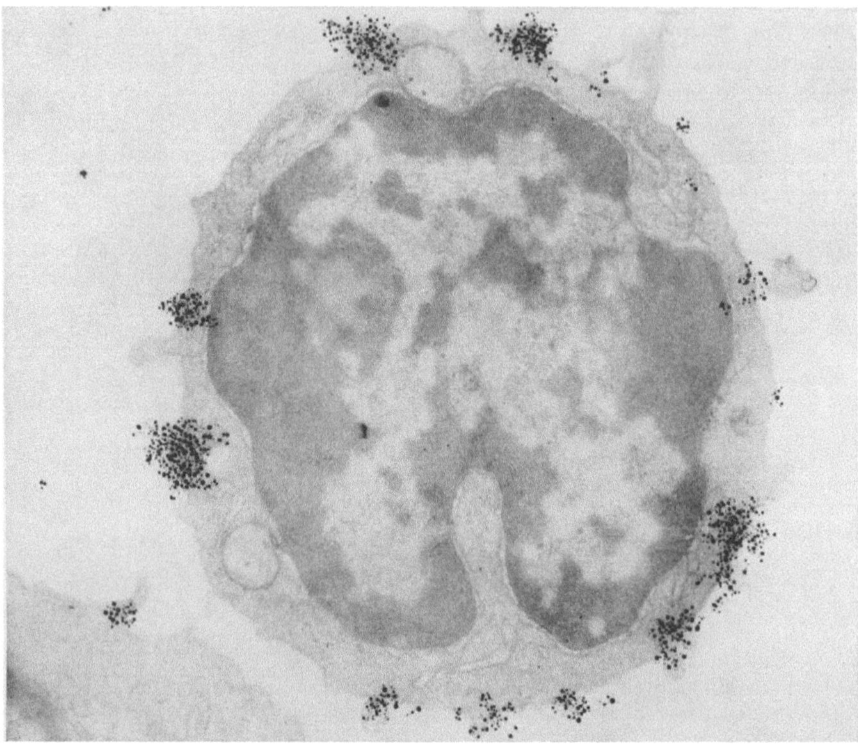

Fig. 1. Electron microscope autoradiograph of a spleen lymphocyte labelled with ^{125}I-haemocyanin. The antigen is present as a series of discrete patches scattered around the cell periphery

membrane. Again, however, the ferritin was present as small collections of molecules in widely scattered and discrete patches (Fig. 2). Some cells were also seen which contained a few silver grains or ferritin molecules apparently within the cell but the significance of this observation is unknown and is under further study.

The peritoneal cavity contained a heterogenous population of cells which included typical macrophages, typical lymphocytes, medium sized mononuclear cells and some granulocytes. A few morphologically typical labelled lymphocytes were seen and these were identical in structure and labelling pattern with the splenic lymphocytes. Most of the labelled "lymphocyte like" cells described by Byrt and Ada [3], however, did not have a typical lymphocytic morphology when viewed in the electron microscope and contained more organelles and a more irregular nucleus. These cells, however, also labelled mainly at the cell surface although some antigen was clearly intracellular. The identity of these cells is uncertain but various data, to be discussed fully elsewhere, suggest that they too are lymphocytic cells rather than monocytic macrophage precursors.

In marked contrast to the lymphoid cells was the behaviour of the peritoneal macrophages. These cells formed a characteristic population and, when they were exposed to the various markers, all the markers were rapidly ingested into lysosome-

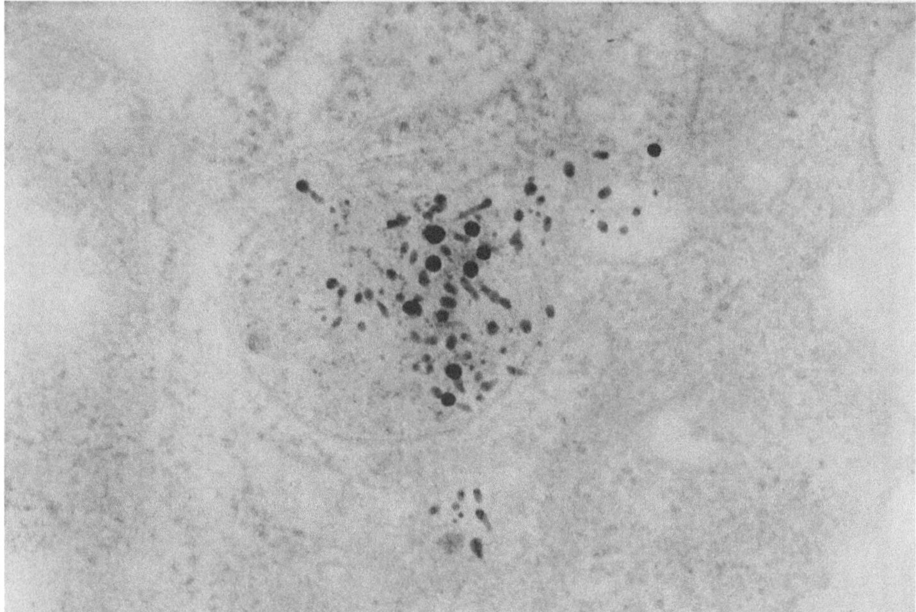

Fig. 2. Portion of a peritoneal lymphocyte showing two patches of ferritin situated just outside the cell membrane. Both patches consist of a few molecules and are separated by an expanse of antigen-free membrane

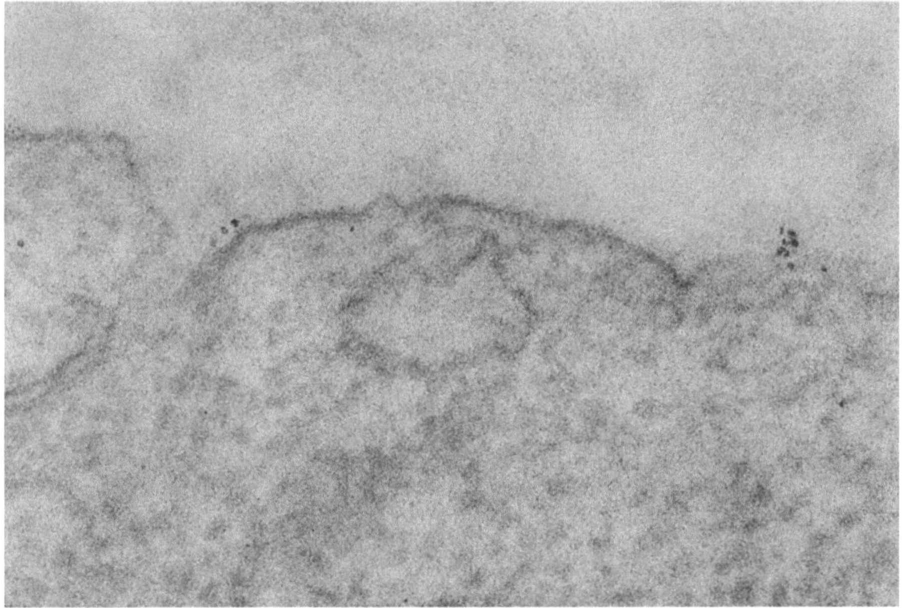

Fig. 3. An electron microscope autoradiograph showing a portion of the cytoplasm of a peritoneal macrophage. Particles of colloidal gold chloride, and ferritin and silver grains from the radio iodinated haemocyanin are all located within and over a membrane-bounded lysosome-like vacuole

like vacuoles (Fig. 3). Within 10 min of exposure most of the particles were intracellular and after 30 min virtually no particles, either immunogens or non-immunogens were seen at the cell surface. The uptake of the particles was by phagocytosis or pinocytosis and all rapidly entered lysosome-like vacuoles. No segregation of the particles occurred within the cell and mixtures of various markers were seen within single lysosomes (Fig. 3). In contrast to the findings of Unanue et al. [6] persistent localization of antigens to the surface of macrophages could not be demonstrated.

Much data is still required and in particular the identity and role of the "peritoneal lymphocyte-like" cells is still in doubt and is under further study. However it has been demonstrated that a small proportion of typical lymphocytes have at their surface isolated and discrete receptor sites which appear to bind antigen specifically. Within the limits of the experimental protocol used in this study, it appears that a single cell can only bind one antigen and that these cells do not appear to bind a small non-immunogenic marker such as colloidal gold. These findings contrast sharply with the apparent non specific intracellular uptake of all the markers by typical macrophages.

Acknowledgements

We thank Mr. John Pye for performing the iodinations and Misses Mary Bravington, Maryla Juchnowski and Marjorie Crawford for skilled technical assistance.

This project was supported by grants from the National Health & Medical Research Council of Australia.

References

1. Warner, N. L., Byrt, Pauline, Ada, G. L.: Nature 226, 942 (1970).
2. Naor, D., Sulitzeanu, D.: Nature 214, 687 (1967).
3. Byrt, P., Ada, G. L.: Immunology 17, 501 (1969).
4. Ada, G. L., Byrt, P.: Nature 222, 1291 (1969).
5. Mandel, T., Byrt, P., Ada, G. L.: Exp. Cell Res. 58, 179 (1969).
6. Unanue, E. R., Cerottini, J. C., Bedford, M.: Nature 222, 1193 (1969).

Mechanisms by which Human Macrophages Resist Intracellular Growth of Listeria Monocytogenes: Studies with a Redox Reagent Active in Leprosy and Experimental Tuberculosis (B 663)*

M. J. CLINE

Introduction

Studies of the role of macrophages in the expression of cell-mediated immunity have revealed that resistance to infections which parasitize the macrophage system can be expressed by means of a heightened resistance of macrophages to the intracellular development of such organisms. Mackaness has shown that this heightened resistance ("acquired cellular resistance" or "cellular immunity") can be generated during delayed hypersensitivity reactions in the infected animal; but in general terms, the role of humoral and cell-mediated mechanisms in these phenomena is not yet fully established. Quantitative investigations of cellular immunity therefore require the development of model systems whereby the microbicidal activities of macrophages can be accurately measured and appropriately manipulated. This paper summarizes one such model system, in which a phenazine derivative, B663, active in murine tuberculosis and human leprosy, enhances the ability of human macrophages to resist intracellular multiplication of *Listeria monocytogenes*.

Methodology

Human blood monocytes were isolated by the technique of BENNETT and COHN, utilizing centrifugation through discontinuous gradients of serum albumin, and differential adherence to glass surfaces. After 7 to 10 days of monolayer culture such cells developed into typical macrophages, exhibiting strong reactions for lysosomal acid hydrolases and active phagocytic ability. The bactericidal activity of macrophage monolayers was assessed after phagocytosis of isotope-labelled *Listeria* by disrupting the cells at suitable intervals and undertaking colony counts of further cultures of liberated *Listeria*. This technique measured killing of intracellular organisms, and was independent of the number of bacteria phagocytized over a wide range.

With this system, the effect of oxygen tension (pO_2) and increased oxygen utilization was tested by means of culturing the infected macrophages in various

---

* Editor's Summary.

partial pressures of oxygen, and by adding B663, which has redox properties and is capable of increasing the generation of hydrogen peroxide and the utilization of oxygen by cells in culture.

Results

It was first found that the killing of *Listeria* by macrophages depended on the oxygen tension of the gas phase in culture: at pO_2 of less than 35 mm Hg the fraction of surviving *Listeria* was greatly increased. The addition of B663 (5×10^{-6} M) to cultures of human macrophages markedly enhanced the killing of *Listeria*, although pre-treatment of the organisms with B663 had no effects on their subsequent handling by macrophages. During exposure of the infected macrophages to B663 hydrogen peroxide accumulated in the suspending medium: this was measured by adding catalase, and recording the release of oxygen with an oxygen electrode. Furthermore, B663 stimulated the uptake of oxygen by the macrophage cultures; and part of this respiratory burst was insensitive to the addition of cyanide. It was therefore concluded that B663 stimulated O_2 consumption via extra-mitochondrial pathways, and that some of this extra O_2 was used for the generation of hydrogen peroxide by the metabolically stimulated macrophages.

Discussion

The question naturally arises of whether enhanced utilisation of oxygen for the generation of hydrogen peroxide by macrophages is relevant to mechanisms of microbicidal activity: for the experiments also showed that the potentiation of killing by B663 required fully aerobic conditions. The mechanisms by which neutrophils kill bacteria are known from studies of cationic proteins with antibacterial activity and from studies of two genetic neutrophil disorders, chronic granulomatous disease of childhood, and neutrophil myeloperoxidase deficiency. It is thought that neutrophils kill bacteria by mechanisms which involve the generation of hydrogen peroxide from molecular oxygen and interaction of H_2O_2 with the enzyme myeloperoxidase; cationic proteins are also thought to play a part. However, macrophages, when mature, have no detectable antibacterial cationic proteins and in the process of maturation they lose their myeloperoxidase activity. It is therefore of interest that neutrophils destroy *Listeria* within four hours, whereas after three hours of macrophage infection, *Listeria* have already begun to replicate within the cells.

The conclusion from this study is that macrophage killing of intracellular bacteria requires oxygen in a form available for conversion to hydrogen peroxide; that this metabolic process involves extra-mitochondrial (cyanide insensitive) pathways; and that the action of the redox agent B663 in enhancing cellular resistance to infection involves activation of similar metabolic pathways by concentrations of the drug (1—2 mg/ml) which occur in human serum during successful chemotherapy of leprosy. The importance of this observation may lie in the demonstration that an "anti-microbial" drug may in fact exert its protective effect by boosting the host defence cell. It is tempting to suggest that similar metabolic processes are involved in the expression of cell-mediated immunological resistance to infections which parasitize macrophages.

The Effect of Cyclophosphamide Treatment on Immunological Competence as Measured by the Mixed Lymphocyte Reaction

M. R. Schwarz

With 2 Figures

Cyclophosphamide, an immunosuppressive agent commonly known as Cytoxan, currently enjoys widespread popularity in medicine [1]. In spite of this, one major drawback to its broader application is the absence of an *in vitro* assay that will assess the immunological status of individuals treated with this drug. Recently, it has been recognized that the mixed lymphocyte reaction (MLR) can detect permanent states of tissue tolerance [2] and can also monitor the temporary immunological depression induced by antilymphocytic serum [3], radiation [4], and thymectomy with or without antilymphocytic serum treatment [5]. Because of these findings, the present study was undertaken to determine if the MLR could detect the immunosuppression induced by cyclophosphamide and if so, whether it could monitor this suppression on a temporal basis.

Materials and Methods

In this study, young, adult rats from the highly inbred Lewis strain, were injected intraperitoneally with 100 mgm/kg of freshly prepared cyclophosphamide (Citoxan^R — Mead Johnson, Evansville, Indiana, USA) or an equivalent volume of saline. At varying times from 1 hour to 7 days thereafter, thoracic duct lymphocytes were obtained from the injected rats by means of a cervical fistula [6]. After counting, a portion of the cells was used to prepare the MLR by combining it with similar cells from the F_1 hybrid of the Lewis and Brown Norway strains (F_1 [Lew$\times$BN]) [7]. In addition, 15—25$\times10^6$ of the cells were used for the normal lymphocyte transfer reaction by injecting them intradermally into the ventral abdominal walls of F_1 (Lew$\times$BN) hybrids [8]. In both the mixed reaction and the transfer reaction, if the small lymphocytes of the Lewis rats were immunologically competent, they responded to the genetically foreign Brown Norway antigens [9] of the F_1 hybrid cells by transforming into blast cells. In contrast, the cells from the F_1 hybrids stimulated the Lewis cells to transform but would not themselves undergo morphological change. To quantitate this transformation, ^{3}H-thymidine was added to the cultures for the final 8 hours of the 72-hour culture period. The amounts of ^{3}H-thymidine incorporated by the cells was then determined by liquid scintillation assay.

Results

Fig. 1 depicts the effect that cyclophosphamide had on the number of cells in the thoracic duct lymph. For ease in comparison, the number of cells in the treated animal has been expressed as a percentage of the number of cells in the saline-injected controls. It may be seen that by 1 hour after administration of cyclophosphamide, a 35—40% reduction in cell number had occurred. By 18—24 hours, the maximum depression of 70—75% was evident. This depression persisted until 7 days when a slight but significant rise was noted. On an absolute scale, the number of cells in the thoracic duct lymph of the saline-treated donors ranged between 72 and 112 million per cc.

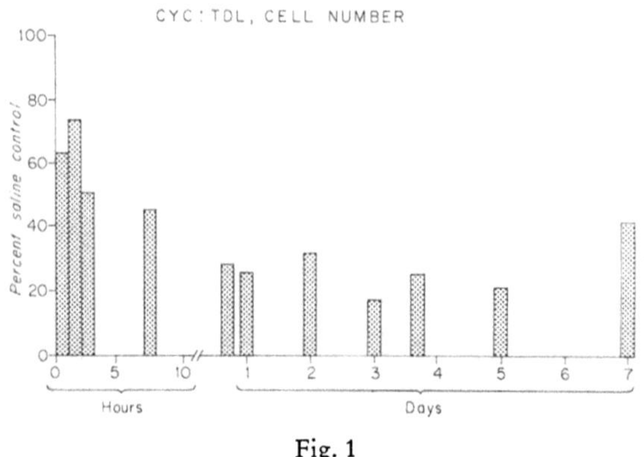

Fig. 1

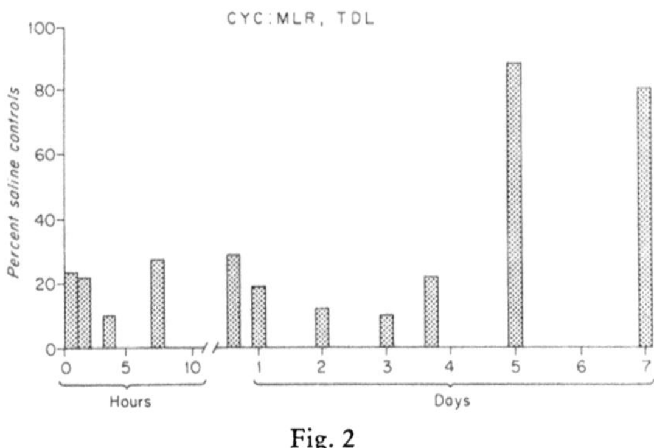

Fig. 2

Fig. 2 depicts the reactivity of thoracic duct cells in the mixed lymphocyte reaction. The amount of ^{3}H-thymidine incorporated by cells from animals treated with cyclophosphamide is expressed as a percentage of the ^{3}H-thymidine uptake by cells from saline-treated donors. As may be seen, the MLR was depressed to 25% of control levels as early as 1 hour after administering cyclophosphamide. This phase of diminished reactivity persisted until 88 hours, when there was a sharp return in cellular competence to near normal levels.

Since the depression could have been due to cyclophosphamide that was attached to the cells at the time they were added to the cultures, 0.5 mgm of cyclophosphamide was added directly to 5 cc mixed cultures initiated with cells from saline-treated donors. Cultures prepared in this way evidenced only $25.3 \pm 1.3\%$ as much ^{3}H-thymidine uptake as controls without the drug.

The results of the normal lymphocyte transfer studies may be seen in Table 1. It is apparent that cyclophosphamide rendered the thoracic duct cells immunologically incompetent for up to 5 days after injection of the drug. Beginning with 5 days a return of competence was noted by the presence of transfer reactions. It should also be noted that this pattern of depression and recovery of the transfer reactions was very similar to that observed with the MLR.

Table 1. *The influence of cyclophosphamide on the ability of thoracic duct cells to produce the normal lymphocyte transfer reactions*

Interval After CYC	Dose of CYC	Diameter of Reaction Saline	CYC
4 hr	100 mgm/kg	7—9 mm	0 mm
16 hr	100 mgm/kg	7—9 mm	0 mm
24 hr	100 mgm/kg	8—11 mm	0 mm
3 d	100 mgm/kg	7—10 mm	0 mm
5 d	100 mgm/kg	7—10 mm	3—4 mm
7 d	100 mgm/kg	7—10 mm	5—7 mm

Abbrv.: hr=hour; d=day; CYC=cyclophosphamide.

Discussion

Since the MLR could be depressed by adding cyclophosphamide to the cultures, it could be suggested that depression observed with cells from treated animals was due to transfer of the drug to the cultures via the cells. This does not seem likely for two reasons. First, maximum depression was evident 88 hours after administration of the drug. Since cyclophosphamide loses its serum activity by 6 hours after injection [10], the depression at 88 hours could not be due to cyclophosphamide in the media. Secondly, the depression observed *in vitro* was also detected *in vivo* with the normal lymphocyte transfer reactions. If the drug were attached to cells which were used to initiate the transfer reactions, it would most likely have been diluted to such low levels that skin lesions would have developed. Since these lesions were not seen before 5 days, the failure of cells to produce transfer reactions has been interpreted as meaning that the cells were immunologically incompetent. As such, the *in vitro* responses of cells in the mixed reactions must also have reflected the immunological competence of cells and possibly the competence of the entire animal.

Summary

The MLR has been shown to monitor the immunological suppression induced by cyclophosphamide treatment. This suppression is most likely not due to contaminating cyclophosphamide in the cultures and is reflected in a similar depression of the *in vivo* normal lymphocyte transfer reaction. It is suggested, therefore, that the MLR may be useful in monitoring the immunosuppressive activity of cyclophosphamide.

Acknowledgements

This study was supported by USPHS Grant No. AI-07509 from the National Institutes of Health.

References

1. Santos, G. W.: Fed. Proc. **26**, 907 (1969).
2. Schwarz, M. R.: J. exp. Med. **127**, 879 (1968).
3. — Tyler, R. W., Everett, N. B.: Science 160, 1014 (1968).
4. Lamberg, J. D., Schwarz, M. R.: Proc. 4th Leucocyte Culture Conf., Hanover, New Hampshire. Ed.: O. R. McIntyre. Appleton-Century-Crofts 1969.
5. Carlson, L. S., Schwarz, M. R.: Proc. 4th Leucocyte Culture Conf., Hanover, New Hampshire. Ed.: O. R. McIntyre. Appleton-Century-Crofts 1969.
6. Reinhardt, W. O., Li, C. H.: Proc. Soc. exp. Biol. (N.Y.) **58**, 321 (1945).
7. Schwarz, M. R.: Amer. J. Anat. **121**, 559 (1967).
8. Ford, W. L.: Brit. J. exp. Path. **48**, 335 (1967).
9. Billingham, R. E., Silvers, W. K.: Plast. reconstr. Surg. **23**, 399 (1959).
10. Ffoley, G. E., Friedman, O. M., Drolet, B. P.: Cancer Res. **21**, 57 (1961).

Influence of E. Coli L-Asparaginase (EC-2 A-se) on Phytohaemagglutinin (PHA)-Stimulated Human Lymphocytes: Inhibition of the Cytoaggressive Effect[*]

H. Oerkermann, W. D. Hirschmann, K. Schumacher, G. Alzer, G. Uhlenbruck, G. Wintzer, and R. Gross

With 1 Figure

It is well known from the studies of other authors that lymphocytes stimulated with PHA destroy cultures of various cell types. Similarly target cells are destroyed in vitro by lymph node cells derived from specifically immunized animals. It was observed that during the so called "cytotoxic reaction" the stimulated lymphocytes enter into close contact with the target cells which seem to play an important role in this process [1—4]. We prefer to call this reaction "cytoaggressive" rather than "cytotoxic" as long as it is not known exactly whether or not toxic agents indeed are concerned in this process. Besides, the term "cytoaggressive" very well describes the special action of the stimulated lymphocytes which appears from the following.

Using time-lapse cinematography we observed, corresponding to the findings of Ax and coworkers [5], that PHA-stimulated lymphocytes were not only passively attached to the target cells but became very mobile and developed great activity. They started to move quickly around underneath and upon the cells of the monolayer culture as soon as they had been added to the target cell culture and had come into contact with PHA. With fine pseudopodia they touched the surface of the target cells and creeping about they pushed the cytoplasm and the nuclei of the target cells to and fro. Those target cells which had been "attacked" for a while suddenly died owing to a rapid breakdown of the cell, remarkably, without previous morphological alterations. During their cytoaggressive action the PHA-stimulated lymphocytes were transformed into blast-like cells and exhibited mitotic cell divisions.

Non-stimulated lymphocytes were comparatively immobile, they did not "attack" the target cells and were not transformed into blast-like cells.

The mechanism of the cell-destroying action of the stimulated lymphocytes against target cells *in vitro* is not yet understood. Since recent investigations had shown that EC-2 A-se inhibits the transformation of PHA-stimulated lymphocytes into blast-like cells [6—8], we wondered whether or not EC-2 A-se also might influence the cytoaggressiveness of the stimulated lymphocytes.

---

* This study was supported by the "Deutsche Forschungsgemeinschaft".

Human lymphocytes, isolated from the peripheral blood of healthy donors by means of a glass bead column, were added to HeLa cell cultures together with PHA and EC-2 A-se. To avoid any inhibitory effect of EC-2 A-se upon the target cells we used a subline of HeLa cells which had been cultured for several months with increasing doses of EC-2 A-se and which had become resistant to this enzyme preparation. The HeLa cells were labelled with ^{14}C-thymidine before they were distributed to the respective cultures of the experiment. We measured the release of ^{14}C-thymidine from the damaged target cells according to the method of Holm and Perlmann [9] to determine the extent of the cytoaggressive effect. The method was slightly modified. After 48 hours of incubation the experiment was stopped and the release of ^{14}C-thymidine was determined. The nutrient medium of the cultures consisted of 20% autologous serum and 80% TC 199. EC-2 A-se was used in a concentration of 3 U/ml culture medium.

It was shown by the experiments that the release of ^{14}C-thymidine was reduced in cultures which had been treated with EC-2 A-se (Fig. 1).

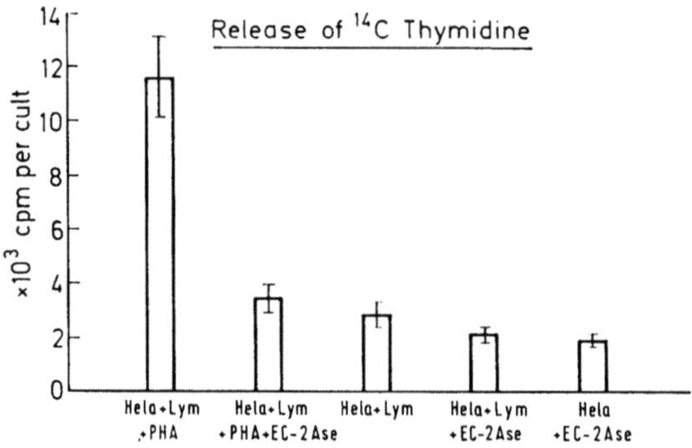

Fig. 1. Mean values of three experiments of the same kind. In all of the tests four cultures were used for each of the five groups

Continuous microscopic observations in phase contrast and time-lapse cinematography of the cultures revealed that, indeed, the cytoaggressive effect of the stimulated lymphocytes was reduced to a minimum. However, and this was an unexpected finding, the typical activity of the lymphocytes was not inhibited by EC-2 A-se. As usual they were moving quickly around and "attacked" the HeLa cells as described above, but the HeLa cells were no longer injured by this action. After 48 hours the monolayer was still intact and the proliferation of the HeLa cells was undisturbed. The lymphocytes, though highly active, were not transformed into blast-like cells and did not exhibit mitotic cell divisions.

To summarize the results, we want to state that EC-2 A-se not only inhibits the blastogenesis of PHA-stimulated lymphocytes but also their cytoaggressiveness. The PHA-induced increased motility of the lymphocytes and their tendency to enter into close contact with the target cells are not affected by EC-2 A-se.

With regard to the mechanism of the cytoaggressive effect, it is shown that this effect apparently cannot be realized by close contact between the lymphocytes and the target cells and by the increased motility of the lymphocytes alone. It must be assumed that this special way of cell destruction requires additional factors to come into play, factors which we do not yet know.

As EC-2 A-se influences the metabolism of certain cell types by depriving them of L-asparagine and/or L-glutamine, it is possible that EC-2 A-se stops the PHA-stimulated lymphocytes from synthesizing certain substances which are additionally necessary to bring about the cytoaggressive effect. How far the synthesis of those substances is connected with the blastic transformation of the stimulated lymphocytes remains to be seen. As the blastic transformation and the cytoaggressive effect are both suppressed by EC-2 A-se, such a connection is certainly conceivable. Finally, it must be considered whether the blastic transformation itself represents the additional factor for the cytoaggressive effect. The stimulated lymphocytes entering into the blastic transformation and preparing cell division have an increased nutritional requirement and this might induce them to develop "parasitic properties" towards the target cells. By withdrawing essential components from the target cells they might cause their destruction — the cytoaggressive effect.

References

1. ROSENAU, W., MOON, H. D.: J. nat. Cancer Inst. **27**, 471 (1961).
2. WILSON, D. B.: J. Cell Comp. Physiol. **62**, 273 (1963).
3. HOLM, G., PERLMANN, P., WERNER, B.: Nature **203**, 841 (1964).
4. MÖLLER, E.: Science **147**, 873 (1965).
5. AX, W., MALCHOW, H., ZEISS, J., FISCHER, H.: Exp. Cell Res. **53**, 108 (1968).
6. ASTALDI, G., BURGIO, G. R., KRC, J., GENOVA, R., ASTALDI, A. A.: Lancet **1969** I, 423.
7. OHNO, R., ANDERSON, M. D.: Proc. Amer. Ass. Cancer Res. **10**, 66 (1969).
8. OERKERMANN, H., HIRSCHMANN, W. D.: Proc. 6th Internat. Congr. Chemother., Tokyo, 1969 (in press).
9. HOLM, G., PERLMANN, P.: Nature **207**, 818 (1965).

Mitotic and Chromosomal Abnormalities Induced by Disrupted Lymphocytes Obtained from Patients with Autoimmune Disorders and Lymphoid Malignancies

T. Hoshino, S. Kawasaki, S. Itani, S. Nakayama, and M. Fukase

With 3 Figures

Introduction

There is evidence indicating an association of autoimmune diseases with chromosomal abnormalities. For instance, the prevalence of chronic thyroiditis is reported to be higher in Down's syndrome [1] and gonadal dysgenesis [2], and positive circulating thyroid autoantibodies have been found in high frequency in the family members of such patients [3]. Patients with a sex-linked congenital immune deficiency syndrome and relatives of these subjects are also highly prone to autoimmune disorders [4]. This suggested to us that both somatic and sex chromosomal abnormalities of congenital origin are in some way responsible for the pathogenesis of autoimmune diseases. In fact, our previous study disclosed such various chromosomal inconsistencies as hyperploidy, dicentrics, minute chromosomes and some diversities in the shape of large-sized chromosomes in lymphocytes of patients with systemic lupus erythematosus [5]. Rhodes reported a possible sex-linkage in the serum level of IgM which is controlled by genes located on the X-chromosomes [6].

On the other hand, Fialkow reported that lymphocyte extracts prepared from patients with chronic thyroiditis or systemic lupus were capable of inducing a dose-dependent high frequency of hyperploid mitosis, chromosomal breakage and rearrangement in allogeneic fibroblasts *in vitro* [7, 8]. He suggested that cell-bound factors, possibly antibodies contained in the lymphocytes, were at least responsible for such effects, and in part selfrecognizing mechanisms were involved in this reaction.

In order to investigate the presence of such cell-bound factors of lymphocytes in systemic autoimmune diseases and malignant lymphoma (in which autoimmunity is believed to be closely related to its pathogenesis), and to study the dynamic effects of such factors on cell division and chromosomal constitution, disrupted lymphocytes of these patients were tested on viable normal lymphocytes cultured with phytohemagglutinin.

Materials and Methods

Circulating lymphocytes were collected from heparinized venous blood by means of a glass-cotton column method under sterile conditions, and were washed twice in TC-199. The final cell suspension contained 85 to 95% lymphocytes. The lymphocyte population thus collected from patients with various autoimmune diseases and malignant lymphoma, or from control normal donors, were disrupted by freezing and thawing 10 times in TC-199 free of serum, followed by heat inactivation at 56° C for 30 min. These disrupted lymphocytes were added directly to the viable washed lymphocyte suspension obtained from a normal man by the same glass-cotton column procedure, and cultured in a mixture of TC-199 and bovine serum in the presence of phytohemagglutinin at 37° C for 3 days. After colchicine treatment, the cultured cells were harvested for chromosomal preparation by the conventional method. Under a microscope, 250 to 500 metaphases were examined for each case, and cells with hyperploid chromosomes more than 3N were scored as a percentage of the total mitoses. Precise karyotype analysis was performed on photographic plates of 10 to 40 randomly selected mitoses of every culture.

Results

As Fig. 1 shows, the frequency of hyperloid mitosis over 3N observed in allogeneic lymphocytes of a normal man was significantly increased when the disrupted lymphocytes from patients with systemic lupus erythematosus (SLE), progressive

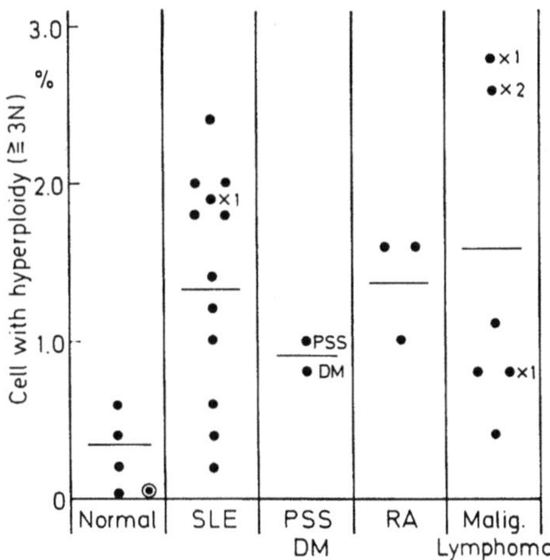

Fig. 1. Hyperploidy effect of allogeneic disrupted lymphocytes from patients and normal subjects on cultured normal lymphocytes with PHA. ⊙ Recipients' lymphocytes per se; $\times_1$ Positive Coombs test; $\times_2$ Monoclonal gammopathy

systemic sclerosis (PSS), dermatomyositis (DM), rheumatoid arthritis (RA) and malignant lymphoma were added to the culture, as compared with those from normal donors. The hyperploidy effect of disrupted lymphocytes obtained from these patients seemed unlikely to be dependent only on the dose added to the culture, but correlated to some extent, with the severity of the disease and with the presence of associated autoantibodies of the donors.

The karyotype analysis demonstrated various forms of chromosomal abnormalities in the metaphase of allogeneic normal lymphocytes cultured with disrupted lymphocytes obtained from these patients (test culture). As Fig. 2 illustrates, such abnormalities as hyperdiploidy, rearrangement and translocation were found in about 10%, 15% and 5%, respectively, in the cultures with disrupted lymphocytes from SLE, RA and DM, and almost similar numbers from malignant lymphoma, while such abnormalities were not seen or rarely observed in the control cultures with disrupted lymphocytes of normal subjects. The other chromosomal aberrations such as deletion and acentric fragment were more frequently scored even in the controls, but the test culture showed 2 to 3 times higher frequencies than the control. Thus, cells with normal karyotype scored 60% in the test cultures and 93% in the control culture.

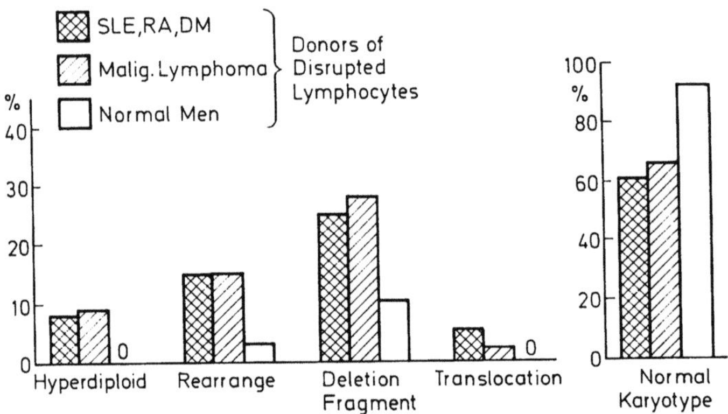

Fig. 2. Chromosome changes in lymphocytes from a normal man cultured with PHA and allogeneic disrupted lymphocytes

The distribution of numerical and structural abnormalities by chromosome groups showed somewhat singular patterns. Although trisomy, rearrangement, deletion and translocation were scattered in every group, it was noteworthy that A-, D- and E-group chromosomes contained more abnormalities than the other groups. Furthermore, new abnormal cell clones with a deletion of the short arm in one of E chromosomes, with E-trisomy and a deletion of the short arm in each one of D- and E-chromosomes have developed in cultures with disrupted lymphocytes from 2 cases of SLE, and a case of malignant lymphoma, respectively.

Fig. 3 shows several representative examples of abnormal karyotypes observed in the test culture: A shows cells with hyperdiploid chromosomes, B gives two karyotypes with rearrangements, C shows two karyotypes with a deletion of short arm of E-18 chromosome associated with other inconsistent structural abnormalities, and D demonstrates dicentric chromosome and reciprocal translocation.

A
C-106-B
47,XY
?G+
B
C-112-B
46,X?Y
A+,G-
C-112-A(5)
47,XY
2+
C-114-A
46,XY
A+,C-
C-114-A
46,XY
Dp-,18p-
C-103 岡本(1)
45,XY,4-,16-,t(4q 16p)+
C
C-114-A
46,?XY
?A+,C-,18p-
D
C-103 岡本(1)
O+ 46,XY,t(12p+;19q-)

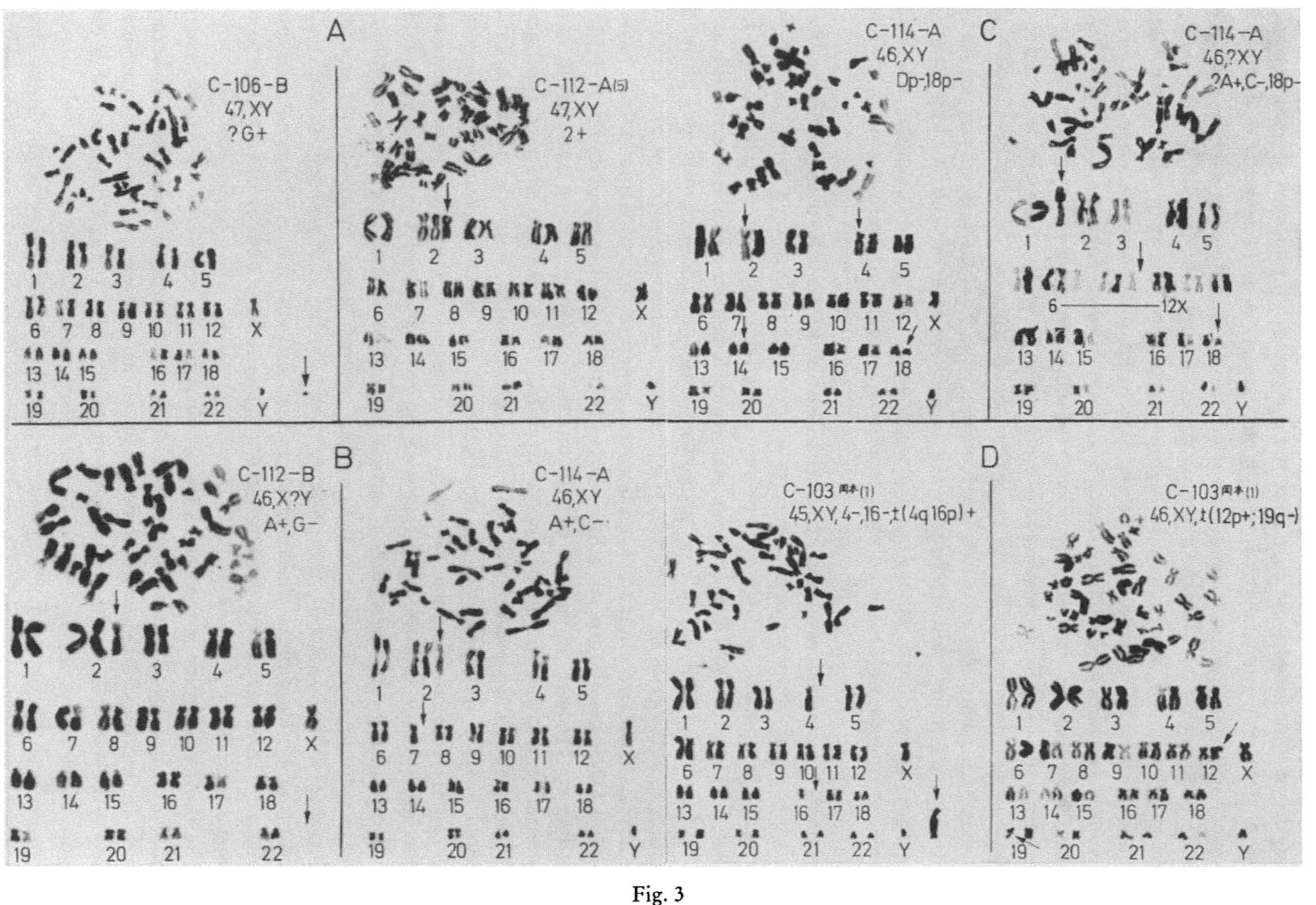

Fig. 3

Discussion

The results of experiments indicate that the disrupted lymphocytes of patients with SLE, PSS, DM, RA and malignant lymphoma contain a certain factor or factors in their subcellular fraction producing abnormalities in cell division and in the chromosomal constitution of allogeneic lymphocytes *in vitro*. Discussion on the pathogenetic mechanism of the factors is highly speculative but it is clear that histoincompatibility could not account for the significant differences between the effects of disrupted lymphocytes from patients and from normal donors.

First, the effects of disrupted lymphocytes might be simply the response to antibodies contained in patients' sensitized lymphocytes [7] with consequent occurrence of cell fusion, non-disjunction, errors in chromosomal distribution and breakage. Cell fusion has been demonstrated when lymphocytes from animals reciprocally sensitized against each other by skin grafting were mixed together in culture [9]. Marked increase in chromosomal breakage, rearrangement, bridge and lagging has been reported in human fibroblast culture treated with extracts of allogeneic lymphocytes [10].

Secondly, some cell products other than antibody may lead to certain mitotic and chromosomal abnormalities. There is evidence that sensitized lymphocytes can have both cytopathic and growth-promoting effects on nonsensitized cells. For instance, RNA extracted from lymphocytes which had been stimulated either *in vitro* [11] or *in vivo* [12] is capable of promoting transformation, mitosis and antibody formation in autologous or allogeneic lymphocytes, respectively. Maini also reported that antigen-activated human lymphocytes generate a mitogenic factor which stimulates DNA metabolism of allogeneic and autologous human lymphocytes [13]. According to Frenster, a variety of substances, including histone and RNA, bind preferentially to either single- or double-stranded DNA and the effect of the ligand on RNA synthesis at preselected gene loci is correlated with the form of DNA preferred [14]. If such processes are applicable to the effects of disrupted allogeneic lymphocytes from autoimmune diseases, the factors in the lymphocytes of these patients might cause mitotic imbalance leading to hyperploidy and bind to a DNA strand, producing chromosomal abnormalities. The circulating lymphocytes in Hodgkin's disease are known to differ from normal blood in amount of actively synthesizing DNA and cell morphology and similar changes are found under conditions of krown antigen challenge, including SLE and RA [15], so that disrupted lymphocytes from malignant lymphoma cases might have similar effects as in autoimmune diseases.

The third possibility is the relevance of virus to the results of our study. Harris has shown that cells of human origin could be fused together into artificial heterokaryons or multinucleated cells with nuclei of diverse origins in the experiment producing hybrid cells in the presence of certain viruses [16]. Chromosomal breakage and translocation are known to be frequently produced by a viral infection. If the lymphocytes of our patients carried viruses, then virus release might induce both hyperploidy and chromosomal effects. Mellors has demonstrated virus-like particles in cells of NZB mice with positive antiglobulin tests [17] and in cells of Swiss mice with hemolytic and renal diseases which had been neonatally given cell-free filtrates prepared from NZB/Bl mice [18].

Our suggestion views new abnormal lymphocyte clones as developing due to effects of disrupted lymphocytes which *in vivo* may generate proliferation of "forbidden clones" of lymphocytes carrying cell-bound autoantibodies.

Summary

1. Disrupted circulating lymphocytes from patients with SLE, PSS, DM and malignant lymphoma were added to the culture with PHA of viable allogeneic lymphocytes from a normal man.

2. Hyperploid mitosis over 3N in metaphase of allogeneic lymphocytes was significantly more frequent in culture with disrupted lymphocytes from these patients than from normal donors.

3. Various chromosomal abnormalities including hyperdiploidy, rearrangement, translocation and breakage were frequently observed in the cultures from these patients.

References

1. MELLON, J. P., et al.: J. ment. Defic. Res. 7, 31 (1963).
2. WILLIAMS, E. D., et al.: New Engl. J. Med. 270, 805 (1964).
3. FIALKOW, P. J., in: Progress in Medical Genetics. Ed.: A. G. STEINBERG. New York: Grune and Stratton 1969, p. 117.
4. FUNDENBERG, H. H., et al.: Med. Clin. N. Amer. 49, 1533 (1965).
5. ITANI, S.: Acta haemat. jap. (in press).
6. RHODES, K., et al.: Brit. med. J. 1969 II, 439.
7. FIALKOW, P. J.: Amer. J. hum. Genet. 18, 93 (1966).
8. — et al.: Nature 211, 713 (1966).
9. OHNO, S., in: The Wistar Institute Symposium Monograph No. 3. Philadelphia: Wistar Institute Press 1965, p. 70.
10. FIALKOW, P. J.: Science 155, 1676 (1967).
11. HASHEM, N.: Science 150, 1460 (1965).
12. COHEN, E. P.: Nature 214, 462 (1967).
13. MAINI, R. N., et al.: Nature 224, 43 (1969).
14. FRENSTER, J. H.: Nature 208, 1093 (1965).
15. CROWTHER, D.: Brit. med. J. 1969 II, 473.
16. HARRIS, H., et al.: Nature 205, 640 (1965).
17. MELLORS, R. C., et al.: J. exp. Med. 124, 1031 (1966).
18. — et al.: J. exp. Med. 126, 53 (1967).

Migration Inhibitory Factor and Mitogenic Factor Produced by Antigen-Stimulated Human Lymphocytes

H.-D. Flad and G. Hochapfel

With 2 Figures

Sensitized human lymphocytes generate *in vitro* a variety of humoral factors when exposed to the specific antigen [1—5]. The present study deals with two of these factors, migration inhibitory factor and mitogenic factor, and their correlation with delayed skin reactions of the lymphocyte donor. Furthermore, preliminary results will be presented indicating that lymphocytes of patients with impaired cell- mediated immunity may be transformed by mitogenic factor.

Lymphocytes from Mantoux-sensitive donors were cultured at 10^7 cells/ml in MEM Eagle (80%)-AB serum 20% containing l-glutamine, Penicillin (100 I.U./ml) and Streptomycin (50 µg/ml). To half of the culture bottles 10 µg/ml tuberculin (PPD, Weybridge) was added. 72 hours later cell-free supernatants were harvested and passed through Millipore filters (0.45 µ). Supernatants of cultures not incubated with PPD were "reconstituted" with PPD (10 µg/ml). All supernatants were supplemented with 15% normal inactivated (56° C, 30 minutes) guinea-pig serum and added in various proportions to Mackaness-type chambers containing capillary tubes filled with peritoneal exudate cells from normal guinea pigs. 24 hours later the inhibition of macrophage migration was determined as described previously [1, 6].

The results show that lymphocytes of 8 Mantoux-sensitive donors produced migration inhibitory factor (MIF) which inhibited the migration of macrophages by more than 25%, of 2 donors by 20—25% and of 3 donors by less than 20% (Table 1). There was no production of MIF by lymphocytes from 3 PPD-negative subjects.

The finding that culture supernatants of some Mantoux-sensitive subjects were not inhibitory, although the DNA synthesis of lymphocytes from these donors was strongly stimulated by PPD, suggested that MIF production and blast transformation might be independent mechanisms. This finding suggested that blast transformation might be associated with the production of a mitogenic factor recently described [3, 4]. Therefore, PPD-preincubated and PPD-reconstituted supernatants were added to triplicates of secondary cultures of lymphocytes from Mantoux-negative subjects. The cultures were maintained at 37° C in an atmosphere of 5% CO_2 in air for 6 days. Lymphocyte stimulation was determined by liquid scintillation counting of uptake of 2-^{14}C-thymidine added 16 hours before harvesting the cultures. Fig. 1 gives an example of mitogenic activity when different volumes of supernatants of

Table 1

$$\text{Migration inhibition (\%)} = 100 - \frac{\text{Area of migration with antigen}}{\text{Area of migration with antigen added afterwards}} \times 100$$

Inhibition of migration (%) of normal guinea pig P. E. cells by lymphocyte culture supernatants from Mantoux-positive and Mantoux-negative subjects

| | Migration inhibition | | |
	+ >(25%)	(+) (20—25%)	— <(20%)
Mantoux-positive : 13	8	2	3
Mantoux-negative : 3	—	—	3

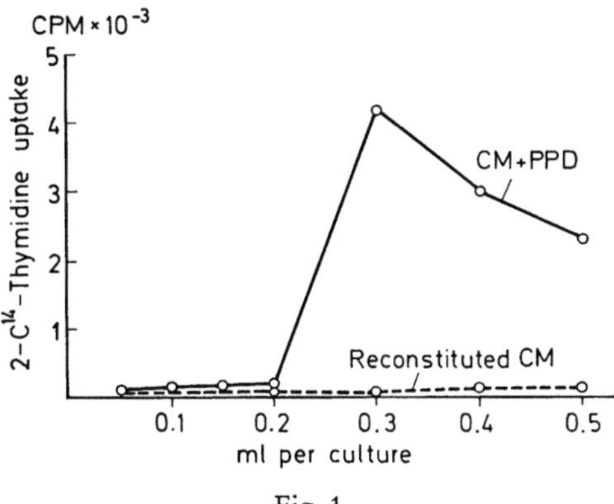

Fig. 1

primary cultures were added to secondary cultures of non-sensitized cells. There was an optimal concentration of preincubated supernatant for stimulation, whereas supernatant reconstituted with PPD did not stimulate. Furthermore, mitogenic factor was released only in the presence of the specific antigen (PPD) and not in the presence of an unrelated antigen (BSA) (Fig. 2). Its activity is maximal at 6 days (Fig. 2).

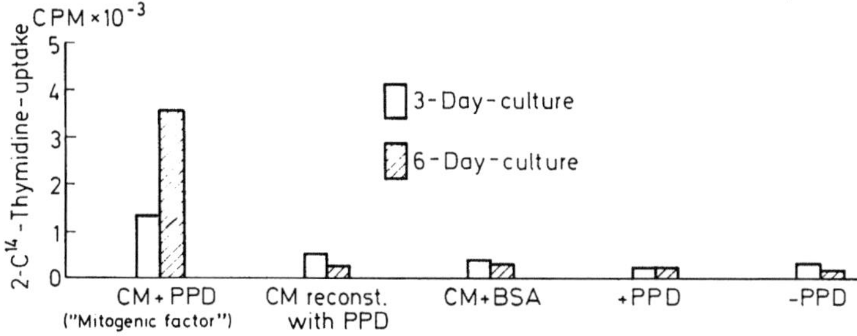

Fig. 2

In a series of experiments, supernatants of lymphocyte cultures from Mantoux-sensitive subjects were examined for both migration inhibitory activity and mitogenic activity (Table 2). Table 2 shows that supernatants from cultures of donors 1—3 were not inhibitory but exhibited mitogenic activity (expressed as C.P.M. obtained with preincubated supernatants minus C.P.M. obtained with reconstituted supernatants, P minus R).

Table 2. *Lack of correlation between migration inhibitory and mitogenic activity (P-R) of lymphocyte cultures supernatants from normal Mantoux-positive donors*

Donor	Mantoux sensitivity (mm)	Migration inhibition tested on normal guinea pig P. E. cells (%)	2-^{14}C-thymidine uptake of lymphocyte cultures from Mantoux-negative persons +PPD (CPM)	P-R (CPM)
J. F.	40×30	13	188	4055
K. M.-H.	20×20	17	62	1505
F. R.	15×15	1	1186	9194
H. F.	15×15	59	135	2832
D. H.	15×15	39	1129	4574

Supernatants from cultures of donors 4 and 5 were both inhibitor and mitogenic. These observations support previous observations [4] suggesting that MIF and mitogenic factor are different biological effector molecules.

The question was raised whether mitogenic factor may also be able to stimulate lymphocytes from patients with impaired cell-mediated immunity to tuberculin. Consequently, supernatants of lymphocyte cultures from Mantoux-sensitive donors were tested in secondary cultures of lymphocytes of patients with chronic lymphocytic leukemia. Table 3 shows that lymphocytes of 3 patients who had low peripheral lymphocyte counts (6000—12000 cells/µl) were able to be stimulated by both PHA (72 hours after onset of culture) and moderately by mitogenic factor. In contrast, lymphocytes of one patient with a high peripheral lymphocyte count (200000 cells/µl) were not stimulated by mitogenic factor and only slightly by PHA. It may be

Table 3. *Mitogenic activity of lymphocyte culture supernatants from normal Mantoux sensitive donors tested in lymphocyte cultures from patients with CLL*

Pat. with CLL	Mantoux sensitivity	Peripheral leucocyte count	2-^{14}C-thymidine uptake of lymphocyte cultures (CPM/culture)			
			+PHA	+PPD	Control	P-R
E. S.	1 : 10²	12600	30432	6931	665	3453
H. SCH.	neg.	6200	21075	129	123	364
M. R.	neg.	8100	24450	163	182	829
G. G.	neg.	200000	1337	132	111	3

concluded from these observations that in patients with low cell counts there might be a small proportion of possibly normal, non-sensitized lymphocytes susceptible to PHA-induced and mitogenic factor-induced stimulation, whereas in patients with high cell counts this populations is absent.

Acknowledgements

The technical assistance of Mrs. A. von Neubeck and Mrs. J. Flad is gratefully acknowledged.

Summary

PPD-stimulated lymphocytes from Mantoux-positive subjects are transformed into blast cells and generate *in vitro* mitogenic factor without migration inhibitory factor being detected. Preliminary results indicate that lymphocytes from patients with chronic lymphocyte leukemia may be stimulated by mitogenic factor. It is suggested that this stimulation depends on the presence of a proportion of normal lymphocytes within the population of leukemic cells.

References

1. Thor, D. E., Jureziz, R. E., Veach, S. R., Miller, E., Dray, S.: Nature 219, 755 (1968).
2. Granger, G. A., Shacks, S. J., Williams, T. W., Kolb, W. P.: Nature 221, 1155 (1969).
3. Maini, R. N., Bryceson, A. D. M., Wolstencroft, R. A., Dumonde, D. C.: Nature 224, 42 (1969).
4. Valentine, F. T., Lawrence, H. S.: Science 165, 1014 (1969).
5. Flad, H.-D., Hochapfel, G.: Europ. J. clin. Invest. (abstract) 1 (1970).
6. David, J. R., Al-Askari, S., Lawrence, H. S., Thomas, L.: J. Immunol. 93, 264 (1964).

In vitro Studies on Human Lymphocyte Factors of Sensitized Lymphocytes

H. M. Dosch, K. Havemann, H. Malchow, C. P. Sodomann, and M. Schmidt

With 5 Figures

It has been shown that sensitized lymphocytes after exposure to antigen generate certain soluble factors which seem to be humoral mediators of cellular immunity.

Evidence for release of mitogenic activity during interaction of sensitized lymphocytes with specific antigen has been given by Dumonde and coworkers. These factors seem to work independently from transplantation antigens and from humoral antibodies on non-sensitized lymphocytes.

Our special interest was related to the production of mitogenic factor by human lymphocytes. We used the system described [1], see Table 1.

Table 1. *Culture assay for testing mitogenic factor and inhibiting factor.* (Dumonde et al., 1969)

Primary culture (3 days)	Secondary culture (5 days)
Tuberculin sensitized lymphocytes (MT10^{-3}-10^{-5}+) 30×10^6/10 ml	Autologous and homologous tuberculin sensitized and non sensitized lymphocytes 3×10^6/4 ml
a) preincubated = tuberculin (0.5—60 µg/ml) at start of culture	
b) reconstituted = tuberculin (same amount) control after 3 days of culture	a) and preincubated supernatants (0, 1 — 1, 0 ml)
cpm/µg DNA preincubated — cpm µg DNA reconstituted	b) and reconstituted supernatants (same amount)
a) positive difference = mitogenic factor	
b) negative difference = inhibiting factor	

Sensitized lymphocytes were cultured in the presence of antigen whereas control-cultures were grown without antigen. Supernatants were removed after three days and the controls were reconstituted with antigen. Thereafter both supernatants contained the same amount of antigen. These supernatants were transferred to secondary cultures consisting of autologous or homologous sensitized or non-sensitized cells.

DNA-synthesis which was stimulated in the control culture with reconstituted supernatant was taken as 100%. The effect of preincubated supernatants was expressed as % of these controls.

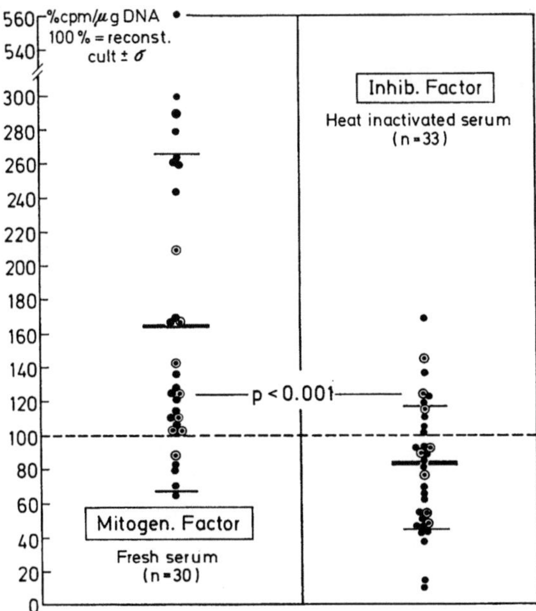

Fig. 1. Response of preincubated in 0/o of reconstituted cultures to tuberculin

The results obtained are plotted in Fig. 1.

If secondary cultures were grown in presence of fresh, autologous serum, the antigen preincubated supernatants caused higher DNA-stimulation than the antigen reconstituted culture supernatants with a mean value of 164⁰/o. These results indicate the production of the mitogenic factor by antigen-stimulated lymphocytes.

If supernatants were tested on autologous or homologous lymphocytes, as indicated by the open (homologous cells) and closed circles (autologous cells), no different response could be observed. This would support the view of other workers that soluble histocompatibility antigens do not play an important role in this reaction [2].

Active supernatants also caused stimulation of the "tuberculin negative" lymphocytes, confirming that the mitogenic factor could be expressed on antigen-insensitive cells ([2].

However, if primary cultures were grown in a medium containing heat-inactivated serum, mitogenic activity of preincubated supernatants was much less apparent. In contrast, in most experiments the activity of these antigen-preincubated supernatants was smaller as compared with the antigen-reconstituted controls. One typical experiment is shown in the Table 2: for the inversion of mitogenic activity to inhibiting activity, the presence of heat-labile serum components is important in primary cultures. The presence of heat-labile proteins in secondary culture is of lower importance, although the effect on mitogenic activity in secondary culture is potentiated. The question arises whether this phenomenon is due to a single factor converted by action of heat-labile serum proteins or whether there are two different factors, production of which was influenced by heat-labile serum components.

Table 2

Heat-labile serum component		REConstituted supernat.		PRE incubated supernat.		PRE — REC	
Primary culture	Secondary	cpm/µg DNA $\bar{x}$		cpm/µg DNA $\bar{x}$			
+	+	5530		1972			
		5344	5330	1779	1974,3	+3556	
		5716		2170			
+	−	2985		1709			
		3078	2985	1840	1706	+1279	
		2892		1573			
−	+	2279		2708			
		2104	2029	4365	3125	−1095,5	
		1799		2304			
		1936					
−	−	1975		2310			
		1811	1725	2884	3252	−2488	
		1389		4562			

In attempt to answer these questions, preincubated and reconstituted supernatants were separated chromatographically on Sephadex G 200 (Fig. 2). Supernatants were taken from primary cultures incubated with 15% heatinactivated serum. All of these revealed inhibiting activity. The fractions were then ultrafiltered, dialyzed, sterile-filtered and tested in secondary cultures without further addition of serum. It could be shown that the supernatants contained two active fractions which differed in molecular weight. An inhibiting factor was found in the macromolecular fraction I and to a minor degree in fraction II. The mitogenic factor was found to be eluted with the albumin-rich fraction.

So far we do not know how these results are related to the above-mentioned inversion of mitogenic activity to inhibiting activity. It may be that a heat-labile serum component is necessary for stabilizing the mitogenic activity or that the inhibiting activity is reduced in the presence of heat-labile serum proteins.

The isolation of mitosis inducing and inhibiting factors is more difficult in the presence of serum proteins in the cultures. We therefore applied a system without serum proteins using PHA as a stimulating agent.

The culture-system used is depicted in Fig. 3. Amounts of PHA inducing maximal DNA-synthesis were added to primary cultures. The supernatants were transferred after cultivation of primary cultures for different periods. Two control systems were used: first, addition of corresponding amounts of PHA to secondary cultures; second, incubation of primary cultures at 4° C. Under these conditions we had factor generation in the primary cultures after certain time intervals. The kinetics of factor production by PHA in 2 experiments are demonstrated in Fig. 4. Each point represents triplicates of secondary cultures grown with supernatants obtained from

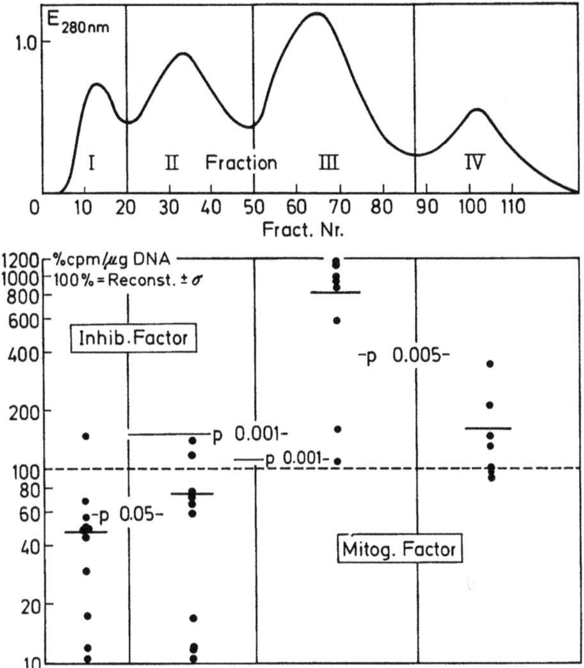

Fig. 2. Chromatography of culture-supernatants on Sephadex G 200

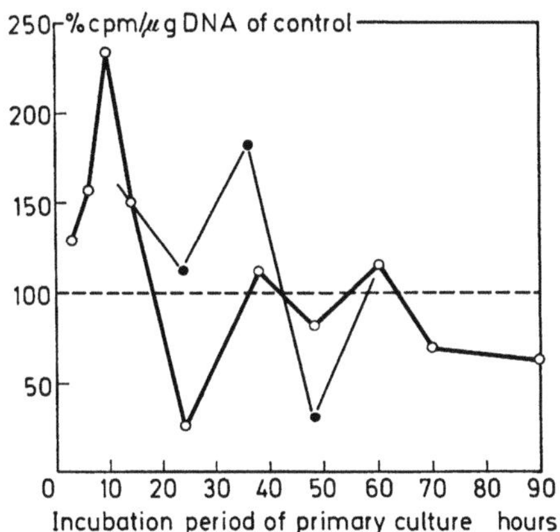

Fig. 3. Factor generation in PHA-cultures w/o serum

primary cultures after different periods of incubation. The secondary culture lasted for 72 hours.

As can be seen, the maximal factor production is found already after 8—12 hours. Later on a decrease and another increase of factor production appears, indicating a rhythm of factor-excretion which is slowing down after longer culture periods.

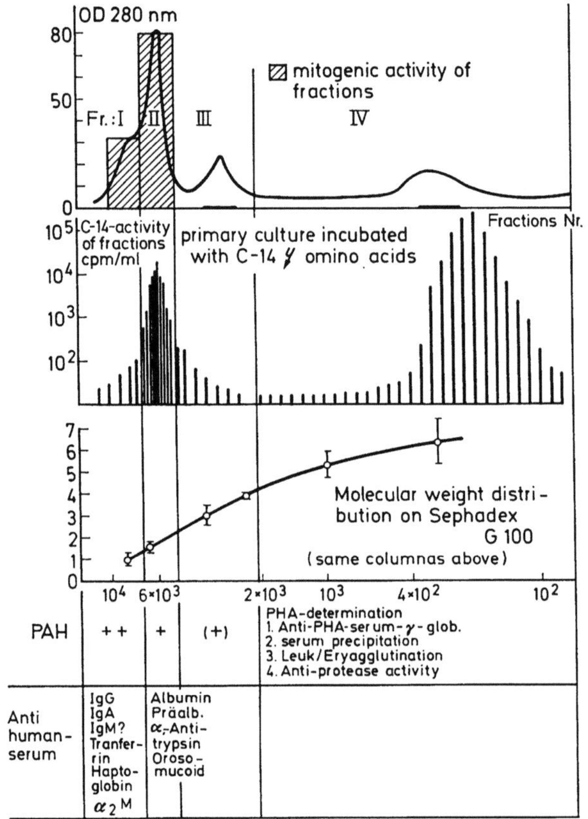

Fig. 4. Mitogenic activity supernatants after different time of incubation with PHA (primary culture with 24 µg/3×10⁶ cells) on secondary culture (72 h). 100⁰/o (6 µg PHA)=maximal PHA activity possibly present in transferred supernatants

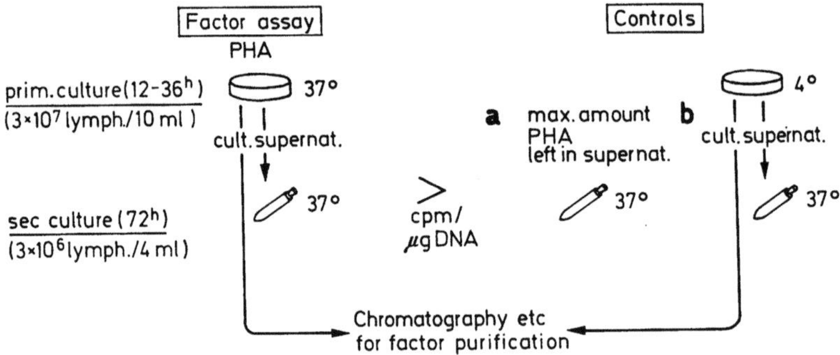

Fig. 5. Exclusion chromatography on Sephadex G 100 of PHA-stimulated primary culture

Preliminary attempts were made to isolate mitogenic activity by chromatography on Sephadex G 100. The distribution of protein present in supernatants is shown in the upper part of the slide. Mitogenic activity was present only in the first 2 fractions. If C-14-labelled amino-acids were added to primary cultures radioactivity

was present in the second major protein peak. The molecular weight of this fraction
was found to be 55 000—65 000 (Fig. 5).

PHA was present in the first macromolecular fraction, but also in the main fraction
although in smaller amounts. An unexpectedly large variety of serum proteins could
be demonstrated by immunelectrophoresis. These were at least in part liberated from
the surface of washed cells present in the cultures.

Summary

1. In a culture-system with antigen and serum proteins, mitogenic factor is
released by human lymphocytes.

2. The mitogenic activity exhibited does not seem to be related to soluble histocompatibility antigens or histocompatibility differences.

3. If heat-inactivated serum was used instead of fresh autologous serum, the
formerly produced mitogenic activity is reversed to an inhibiting one.

4. Mitogenic activity and inhibiting activity seem to be due to different components with different molecular weights.

5. PHA may be used for the production of the mitogenic factor in a serum free
system: this system exhibits a certain rhythm of factor generation.

6. Supernatants from PHA stimulated cultures may be useful for isolation of
the active component.

References

1. DUMONDE, D. C., WOLSTENCROFT, R. A., PANAYI, G. S., MATTHEW, M., MORLEY, J.,
   HOWSON, W. T.: Nature 224, 38 (1969).
2. MAINI, R. N., BRYCESON, A. D. M., WOLSTENCROFT, R. A., DUMONDE, D. C.: Nature 224,
   43 (1969).

The Effect of DEAE-Dextran on Stimulated Human Lymphocytes, with and without "Exogenous" RNA

P. G. RIGBY

Introduction

Diethylaminoethyl dextran (DEAE-Dextran) is a positively charged, long-chain carbohydrate molecule, which has been shown to combine with RNA and to markedly increase the incorporation of RNA into cells. PAGANO and co-workers have shown that the addition of DEAE-Dextran to a tissue culture system increased the incorporation of polio virus RNA into cells 100,000 times [1]. The life span of animals challenged with Ehrlich ascites tumour can be prolonged, as shown from experiments in this laboratory, when DEAE-Dextran is used in the delivery system with "tumour immune" RNA—spleen cell transfers, to a point comparable with actively immunized animals similarly challenged [2]. DEAE-Dextran will also increase the transferability of a mammalian RNA in transplantation immunity at least 1,000 times, using a system of skin allograft rejection, with improvement to the second set time by transfer of "immune" RNA [3]. DEAE-Dextran will increase the stimulation of interferon production when combined with various RNA's including Poly I : C, though no specificity of action has been described in this system [4]. THORLING and LARSEN have shown an inhibitory effect of DEAE-Dextran on tumour growth in several animal systems both *in vivo* and *in vitro* and with reversal by Dextran [5].

Materials and Methods

The DEAE-Dextran was purchased from Pharmacia (Sweden, molecular weight 2 million) and dissolved in normal saline for use. The RNA used in these studies was yeast RNA (Mann Research Laboratories Lot. No. 1491) dissolved in normal saline.

The method of lymphocyte culture was based on that reported by BACH and HIRSCHHORN and later by JOHNSON and RIGBY from this laboratory [6—8]. Heparinized human blood was allowed to sediment at 37° C in screw cap glass tubes for 1—3 hours. Supernatant plasma was removed and 1—2 million cells in plasma were pipetted into tissue culture tubes containing 2 ml of medium (MEM Spinner media, supplemented with 20% fetal calf serum, penicillin (0.1 mg/culture), streptomycin (0.1 mg/culture), and L-Glutamine). The percentage of lymphocytes put into tissue culture (TC) has been improved by careful control of the sedimentation and extraction procedures to approximately 90—95%. The basic suspension was varied by the addition of Phytohemagglutinin, 0.02 ml/ml culture medium (General Biochemicals, Lot. No. 661, 601).

The radioactive counting technique was modeled on that of MAKMAN, DVORKIN, and WHITE and detailed briefly as follows: 3 µCi of tritiated thymidine (specific activity 3 Ci/m mole, SCHWARTZ Biochemical) was added to the tissue culture tubes 68 hours after onset [9]. These were harvested 24 hours later and the reaction was stopped by the addition of 1 ml of cold thymidine (2×10^{-3} M). The cells were washed twice with cold saline (0.9% NaCl), and then the DNA was precipitated with cold 5% trichloracetic acid and the material collected on a 0.45 micron Millipore filter. The filters were dried and dissolved in Bray's scintillant and counted on a Unilux Model II Scintillation counter.

The cell counts were performed by the Chamber technic on the 7th day using Cetrimide in a 1—10 dilution in 1% acetic acid (concentration 5 mg/ml) to avoid the clumped lymphocytes with PHA incubation [10]. Cell cultures were done in triplicate and counts in duplicate. The data in Table 1 is expressed at 4 days as the percent of control tritiated thymidine uptake in terms of counts per minute. On separate culture, the number of cells in tissue culture at 7 days is given and the percent of control indicated.

Results

The number of cells achieved at 7 days in one experiment by the control culture with Phytohemagglutinin was 2.02×10^6 cells, given as 100% in Table 1. This was similar to the result with added Dextran sulfate of molecular weight 5.0×10^5 with Heparin (0.06 ml/TC), or the combination of Heparin and Dextran. DEAE-Dextran, however, with molecular weight 2×10^6, alone at a dosage of 15 µg/TC, resulted in a reduction in the cell number to 1.03×10^6 (51%). The addition of Dextran and Heparin together opposed this suppression, resulting in 1.67×10^6 cells/TC (84%), although Dextran added to DEAE-Dextran invariably precipitated when Heparin was omitted.

The percent of control tritiated thymidine uptake is expressed in the Table 1 and generally parallels the findings with cell counts. Four different experiments were done with DEAE-Dextran at a dose of 15 µg/TC and although these varied from 50—129%, several experiments showed clear depression of uptake or cell counts. The experiments with DEAE-Dextran done at 50 µgm/TC showed 40—68%, also a suppression. This result may vary according to the cell donor and other factors in the tissue culture set up.

The yeast RNA in doses of 1.0 mg or 0.1 mg/2 ml TC added to the DEAE-Dextran did not increase the suppressive effect. It has been shown previously that yeast RNA alone, as well as other kinds of RNA, will suppress antigen or PHA-stimulated normal human lymphocyte transformation [7, 8].

Morphologically, the Wright stain smears of PHA-stimulated normal human lymphocytes with DEAE-Dextran showed gross alterations of the cells, including "ponytail" cytoplasmic streaming, vacuolization, and nuclear fragmentation.

Table 1. *The effect of DEAE-Dextran and RNA on HLT*

Addition to cultures:	Cell Cts. % Cont.	³H-T % Cont.
RNA (1.0 mg/culture)	50	43
	46	31
	76	45
		83
		21
(2.0 mg/culture)		26
RNA (2.0 mg) + DEAE-Dextran (5 µgm/culture)	—	32
DEAE-Dextran (15 µgm/culture)	70	
	68	
	51	
		51
		94
	100	129
DEAE-Dextran (50 µgm/culture)		40
		68
Dextran (15 µgm/culture)	108	111
Dextran (15 µgm/culture) + DEAE-Dextran (15 µgm)		96
Heparin (0.06 ml/culture)	85	85
Heparin + Dextran	86	68
Heparin + DEAE-Dextran	56	91
Heparin + DEAE-Dextran + Dextran	84	83

Discussion

These experiments indicate that DEAE-Dextran will suppress the number of lymphocytes in tissue culture at 7 days, and the percent control uptake of tritiated thymidine
at 4 days in Phytohemagglutinin stimulated human lymphocyte cultures. This effect
was reversed by the combination of Dextran and Heparin; the suppressive effect
was not impressive with Heparin or Dextran alone or together. There was a correlation between cell counts and tritiated thymidine uptake generally. The addition
of DEAE-Dextran to lymphocytes in tissue culture can result in an agglutination
of cells, which could interfere (especially at high doses) in the ordinary conditions
of tissue culture. There may also be variability in the cells from different donors in
relation to the response to DEAE-Dextran.

DEAE-Dextran can be shown to associate with and to change cell surfaces;
presumably related to its positive charge. Thorling and Larsen have indicated that
DEAE-Dextran is probably not taken up into cells, but attaches to both red cells
and white cells (lymphocytes) in an increasing fashion with dose, changing the
migration of such cells [11]. DEAE-Dextran has also been shown to combine with
RNA outside of cells and to influence the incorporation of RNA into cells [1—4].
The mechanism of action of DEAE-Dextran remains unclear in biologic systems
although the addition of this molecule can be shown to change a number of such
cellular phenomenon. Whether changes are related to cell surface phenomenon or to
attachments to molecules such as RNA outside of cells is still open to question.

WEISS et al. and BIERLE et al. have shown that RNA does occur on the cell surface, and thus could conceivably influence intracellular and intercellular activities through activation or attachment [12, 13].

Prior experiments from this laboratory have shown that DEAE-Dextran has an effect on tumor growth when given directly to mice intraperitoneally [14]. THORLING and LARSEN have previously reported studies indicating that the *in vitro* incubation of tumor cells with DEAE-Dextran was very effective in suppressing tumor growth and that the *in vivo* use of DEAE-Dextran also showed significant prolongation of life [5]. These effects were not improved when DEAE-Dextran was incubated with yeast RNA [14]. Prior studies have shown that "tumor immune" RNA extracted from animals immunized against the tumor was effective in prolonging life when delivered in an effective carrier system with DEAE-Dextran [2]. It may be argued that the greater effect with "specific" RNA was improved by the delivery system using DEAE-Dextran, or possibly that the more specific RNA brought the DEAE-Dextran to the tumor cell area.

An effect of DEAE-Dextran on the immune system could also be suggested in this and other systems. The influence of DEAE-Dextran on the suppression of lymphocyte proliferation does not necessarily mean that immune function would be depressed or that other *in vivo* correlations would follow. There is indication that DEAE-Dextran combined with tumor cells increases the immunization potential of killed cells when followed by tumor challenge [14]. Again RNA does not improve this immunization procedure when given prior to the introduction of the live tumor. RNA and Poly I : C given after live tumor challenge preceded by immunization does influence favorably the life span of the animal, though this finding as yet remains unexplained as to mechanisms [14].

The observations indicating an effect of DEAE-Dextran on the lymphocyte in tissue culture may be related to the interaction of oppositely charged molecules at the cell surface, the influence of DEAE-Dextran on intercellular messages related to cell interaction, or possibly on influences within the actively metabolizing cell based on cell surface contact.

Summary

DEAE-Dextran has been shown to inhibit PHA-stimulated human lymphocyte transformation in tissue culture. No effect was noted by Dextran or Heparin alone or by the combination of these two substances. The reversal of this inhibition was, however, noted when Dextran and Heparin were combined with the DEAE-Dextran in tissue culture.

References

1. PAGONO, J. S., McCUTCHAN, J. H., VAHERI, A.: J. Virology 1, 891—897 (1967).
2. RIGBY, P. G.: Nature 221, 968—969 (1969).
3. — Clin. Res. 16, 470 (1968).
4. DIANZANI, F., CANTAGALLI, P., GAGNONI, S., RITA, G.: Proc. Soc. exp. Biol. (N.Y.) 128, 708—710 (1968).

5. Thorling, E. B., Larsen, B.: Acta path. microbiol. scand. 75, 237—246 (1969).
6. Bach, F. H., Hirschhorn, K.: Sem. in Hemat. 2, 68 (1965).
7. Johnson, D. M., Pratt, P. T., Rigby, P. G.: Blood 29, 800—807 (1967).
8. Rigby, P. G., Johnson, D. M.: Acta haemat. (Basel) 42, 94—98 (1969).
9. Makman, M. H., Dvorkin, B., White, A.: J. biol. Chem. 241, 1646 (1966).
10. Stewart, C. C., Ingram, M.: Blood 29, 628 (1967).
11. Thorling, E. B., Larsen, B.: I. Studies of the Erythrocyte Cell Surface (to be Published).
12. Mayhew, E., Weiss, L.: Exp. Cell Res. 50, 441—453 (1968).
13. Beierle, J. W., Allerton, S. E., Bavetta, L. A.: Tenth International Cancer Congress (Abstract) 429, 266 (1970).
14. Rigby, P. G.: Tenth International Cancer Congress (Abstract) 1315, 798 (1970).

Changes of Euchromatin Content in Human Peripheral Lymphocytes under the Influence of Phytohaemagglutinin

P. DRINGS

With 3 Figures

In the last few years there have been many reports on the metabolic stimulation of lymphocytes by phytohaemagglutinin (PHA), an extract from *Phaseolus vulgaris*. PHA causes an increase of DNA, RNA, and protein synthesis in lymphocytes, stimulates their transformation to lymphoblasts, and induces them to undergo mitosis [1, 2, 8, 9, 12, 14]. The transformation of lymphocytes may be regarded as an example of gene activation in mammalian cells [10, 15].

We know that in somatic cells only a certain portion of the whole genetic information is operational. In interphase nuclei all available information is localized in chromatin, which is in an active, diffusely staining state, termed euchromatin. The condensed part of chromatin, heterochromatin, probably contains that part of the genetic information, which is permanently repressed [7]. It remains unknown which mechanism controls the postmitotic differentiation of chromatin.

It is the purpose of the present investigation to report on studies undertaken to find out whether the increased metabolic activity of lymphocytes by PHA is accompanied by an increase of the euchromatin content. Euchromatin and heterochromatin were isolated from nuclei after the method of FRENSTER et al. [5]. We withdrew 100 ml blood (heparinized) from each of 9 patients without haematological diseases. The patients had not received steroids or immunosuppressive and cytostatic agents. The blood was mixed with $6^0/0$ dextran to a final dilution of 4 : 1 [4], and the cells were allowed to settle for 1 hour at 37° C. The supernatant, which contained the leukocytes and the buffy coat, was removed, centrifuged at low speed for 10 min, and resuspended with serum. Polymorphonuclear leukocytes and monocytes were removed with a glass bead column [6]. The suspension of lymphocytes obtained had a purity of 90—100$^0/0$. The erythrocyte/leukocyte ratio was 3 : 1. The lymphocytes were suspended in MEM, which contained 15$^0/0$ fetal calf serum, 100 units penicillin and 100 µg streptomycin/ml. The final cell concentration varied from 1.5 to 2.5×10^6 lymphocytes/ml. We divided the MEM suspension of lymphocytes into two cultures, each of 10 ml volume. To each we added 0.06 ml PHA-M (General Biochemicals Co.) a concentration found optimal in preliminary tests. Physiological saline was added to control cultures. Chromatin fractions were measured at the beginning of the experiment and after 24 hours' incubation.

Cells were allowed to swell in the hypotonic medium described by Frenster. Nuclei were then suspended in 0.25 M sucrose at 0°, carefully agitated for 10 min in an ice bath, and exposed to the Branson sonifier S 75 for 20 seconds. After disruption of the nuclear membrane, the nuclear contents were fractionated by differential centrifugation. As previously shown, after 10 min at 1000 g the first fraction, the so-called heavy fraction, contains predominantly heterochromatin. After 30 min at 3000 g the second fraction, the so-called intermediate fraction, represents a mixture of both eu- and heterochromatin. After 60 min at 78.000 g the third fraction, the so-called light fraction, is composed predominantly of euchromatin.

The chromatin fractions were dissolved in 1 M saline. The DNA content was determined by extraction of nucleic acids from the chromatin fractions [16], and measuring them colorimetrically with the diphenylamine reaction [3]. The DNA content of the different fractions was given as percent of the total.

As shown in Fig. 1, the relative distribution of DNA in the 3 fractions depends on the duration of sonication. Under our experimental conditions however, the

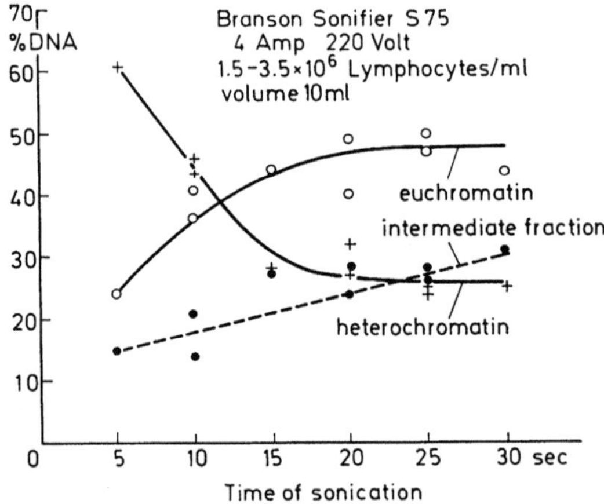

Fig. 1. Percentage of DNA in the euchromatin, heterochromatin and intermediate fraction of nuclei of human peripheral lymphocytes plotted against duration of sonification

relative DNA content of the 3 fractions remained constant after 20 seconds of sonification. The so-called light and heavy nuclear fractions are mainly composed of eu- or heterochromatin respectively. Analytical separations cannot be achieved with Frenster's method. Under strictly standardized conditions, however, relative values may be obtained, and changes in the ratio of eu- to heterochromatin in a given cell type can be analysed [7].

Under the stimulation with PHA the euchromatin of human lymphocytes increased after 24 hours' incubation. Under our experimental conditions 39.5% of DNA was in the euchromatin fraction before stimulation. 24 hours after stimulation the percentage of DNA in the euchromatin fraction had risen to 52.1%. No increase in the euchromatin fraction was found in the 9 control cultures without PHA, since at the beginning of the culture period 43.9% of the total DNA was found in this fraction in contrast to 46.8% after 24 hours. Parallel with the increase of euchromatin, the heterochromatin fraction fell from 33.2% to 24.4% after 24 hours' stimulation with PHA. The heterochromatin fraction remained unchanged in unstimulated cultures with 24.4 and 24% respectively (Fig. 2).

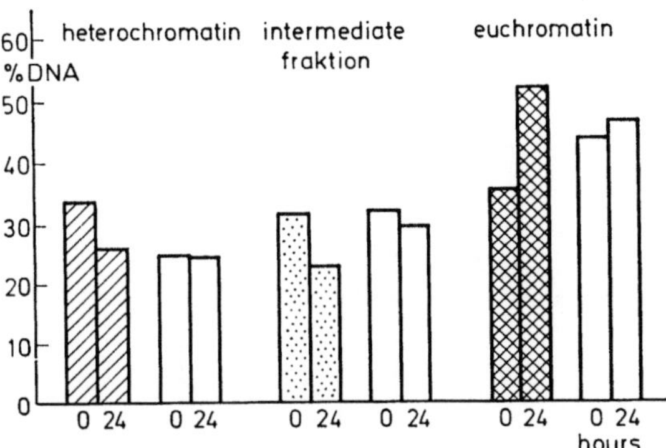

Fig. 2. Percentage of DNA in the different chromatin fractions of nuclei of human peripheral lymphocytes before and after 24 hours of stimulation with PHA. Dark columns represent PHA treated, white columns control cultures

Because the content of DNA in the euchromatin fraction was not independent of that of the intermediate and the heterochromatin fractions, all experimental data were transformed with the linear contrast method. Measurement data were multiplied with a weighting coefficient, the sum of weighting coefficients being 0. The linear contrast of the initial values represented the independent variable x, that of all dependent values the dependent variable y. Thus it was possible to eliminate the influence of different initial values upon values after stimulation in the calculation of the analysis of covariance. The coefficient of regression was +0.36. In other words, if the linear contrast for the independent variable increased or decreased by 1, the value of the dependent contrast changed by approximately one third. After the influence of the independent variable was nullified, the adjusted mean values for the dependent variable could be calculated. The mean value was 0.4666 for the PHA stimulated lymphocytes, and 0.2557 for the controls (Fig. 3). This difference is statistically significant with $\alpha = 0.05$.

The results of our investigation agree with those of MILLNER and HAYHOE [13] obtained by electron microscopy and autoradiography. These authors described a continuous descondensation of heterochromatin during the transformation of lymphocytes. That was paralleled by an increase in the size and numbers of sites with extended chromatin, in which DNA- and RNA-synthesis was found by autoradiography. Decondensation of heterochromatin was maximal in the S-phase. Similiar changes of decondensation of nuclear structure in PHA transformed lymphocytes were shown by IMMAN and COOPER [11]. In this context it may be noted that HIRSCHHORN et al. [10] found an increased primer capacity for nucleotide incorporation into RNA, when nuclei of human lymphocytes were incubated with bacterial RNA polymerase after PHA stimulation. This would imply that more DNA is available for transcription. Stanley et al. [17] observed a selective affinity of PHA for heterochromatin, which they attributed to electrostatic forces. PHA uptake is followed by acetylation of histones which, as Pogo et al. [15] suggested, is in some way involved in derepression of DNA.

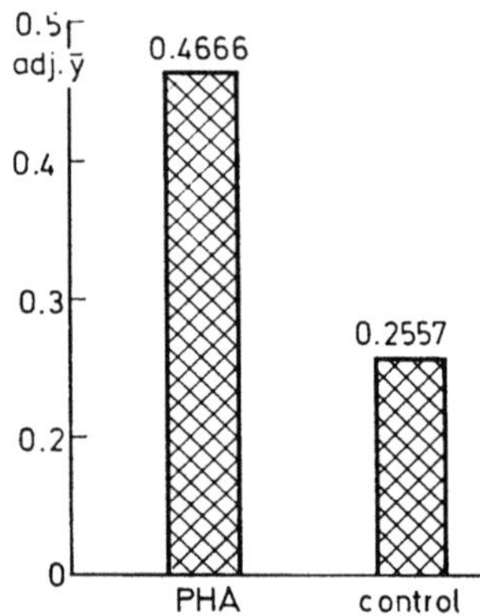

Fig. 3. Analysis of covariance. Adjusted mean values of the dependent variable (euchromatin) of PHA stimulated and control cultures

    In conclusion, our results show that PHA causes euchromatinization in lymphocyte cultures. At present we are studying the influence of steroids and cytostatic agents on this process of euchromatinization.

Acknowledgements

The author is greatly indebted to Dr. Immich (Deutsches Krebsforschungszentrum, Institut für Dokumentation und Statistik) for statistical calculations. He gratefully acknowledges the technical assistance of Mrs. M. Brecht.

References

1. Bach, F., Hirschhorn, K.: Exp. Cell Res. **32**, 592 (1963).
2. Bender, M. A., Prescott, D. M.: Exp. Cell Res. **27**, 221 (1962).
3. Dische, Z.: Mikrochemie **8**, 4 (1930).
4. Engelhardt, A.: Klin. Wschr. **42**, 1141 (1964).
5. Frenster, J. H., Allfrey, V. G., Mirsky, A. E.: Proc. nat. Acad. Sci. (Wash.) **50**, 1026 (1963).
6. Garvin, J. E.: J. exp. Med. **114**, 51 (1961).
7. Harbers, E., Lederer, B., Sandritter, W., Spaar, U.: Virchows Arch. Abt. B Zellpath. **1**, 98 (1968).
8. Hastings, J., Freedman, S., Rendon, O., Cooper, H. L., Hirschhorn, R.: Nature **192**, 1214 (1961).
9. Havemann, K.: Z. ges. exp. Med. **151**, 138 (1969).
10. Hirschhorn, R., Troll, W., Brittinger, G., Weissmann, G.: Nature **222**, 1247 (1969).

11. IMMAN, D. R., COOPER, E. H.: Acta haemat. (Basel) **33**, 257 (1965).
12. McINTYRE, O. R., EBAUGH, F. G., JR.: Blood **19**, 443 (1962).
13. MILNER, G. R., HAYHOE, F. G. J.: Nature **218**, 785 (1968).
14. NOWELL, P. C.: Cancer Res. **20**, 462 (1960).
15. POGO, B. G. T., ALLFREY, V. G., MIRSKY, A. E.: Proc. nat. Acad. Sci. (Wash.) **55**, 805 (1966).
16. SCHNEIDER, W. C.: J. biol. Chem. **161**, 293 (1945).
17. STANLEY, D. A., FRENSTER, J. H., RIGAS, D. A.: J. Cell. Biol. **39**, 129 a (1968).

Inhomogeneity of Peripheral Lymphocytes — Complement Receptor Sites on a Portion of Human Lymphocytes

H. Huber, G. Michlmayr, C. Huber, H. Asamer, and S. D. Douglas

With 3 Figures

The characterization of cell surface receptors on mononuclear cells may give important information on their immunological functions. We and others reported on distinct receptor sites for IgG and the third component of complement present on monocytes and macrophages [3, 4, 6, 7]. Recently immunoglobulin determinants on certain lymphocytes have been demonstrated by several investigators [2, 10, 14]. In order to further assess receptor sites on lymphocytes, the reactivity of normal cells, those separated by density gradients and of cells from patients with chronic lymphocytic leukaemia were tested for the presence of membrane receptors for antigen-antibody-complement complexes. A certain correlation between this sub-population of lymphocytes and those with immunoglobulin determinants on their membrane was observed.

Lymphocytes were isolated from the peripheral blood of 25 normal donors and of 16 patients with chronic lymphocytic leukaemia by filtration through nylon wool. Receptor sites were assessed by their capacity to bind red cells coated with complement (C'). Those were prepared by incubating sheep red cells with appropriate dilutions of rabbit anti-Forssmann antiserum and fresh human serum as a source of C'. In other experiments a homologous system was employed using human red cells sensitized with a typical cold agglutinin of high titer. Control preparations included unsensitized red cells and erythrocytes, which were incubated with antiserum in the absence of C'. A fractionation of lymphocytes according to their density was obtained by centrifugation in a discontinuous albumin gradient [11, 13]. In parallel, experiments on the mouse were performed and lymphocytes obtained from their spleens were assessed for receptor activity. Simultaneously, lymphocytes with immunoglobulin determinants were evaluated in the mouse in a cytotoxic assay by incubating the cells with anti-kappa antiserum, kindly provided by Dr Hans Wigzell. In humans, the lymphocytes with kappa determinants were counted after incubation with a rabbit anti-kappa antiserum and after subsequent labelling with fluorescent anti-rabbit-immunoglobulin antiserum.

Red cells coated with human C' formed rosettes around a significant percentage of blood lymphocytes obtained from normal donors. In the homologous system the percentage of rosette-forming lymphocytes averaged 12% ($\pm$ 2.2%); these experiments were performed at room temperature. In the heterologous system at 37° an average of 20% (±1.4% of lymphocytes were positive. When lymphocytes were incubated with human or sheep red cells alone, rosette formation was an unusual finding (0.25%, 0.1%). This was also true, if red cell-antibody complexes without C' were tested (0.25%, 0.4%).

Red cells were coated with various dilutions of C' and were subsequently added to lymphocytes. With less C on the red cells, the percentage of reactive cells decreased, indicating that the number of lymphocytes with rosettes was related to the amount of C' bound to the red cells (Fig. 1).

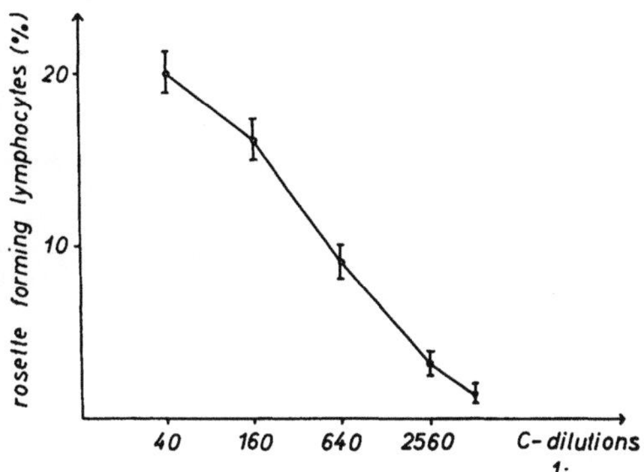

Fig. 1. Percentage of receptor positive lymphocytes related to the amount of complement added

By centrifugation in a discontinuous bovine serum albumin gradient lymphocytes of normal donors were separated into fractions of different density. Five discrete bands of cells were obtained. The percentage of C'-reactive lymphocytes differed markedly between these fractions. The cells on the interphases of albumin of lower concentrations (up to 26%) contained the highest percentage of lymphocytes with C' receptor activity, whereas those in the pellet were almost unreactive.

We then performed electron microscopic studies on receptor positive lymphocytes without and after enrichment of rosette-forming cells in a density gradient. On some cells a very intimate contact between the lymphocyte membrane and the immune complexes was observed. Measurements on these cells revealed a distance of less than 100 Å between both membranes. Reactive cells were almost exclusively small lymphocytes, but on morphological terms distinct differences between receptor positive and negative cells have not so far been observed (Fig. 2).

In order to further characterize lymphocytes with C' receptors, we then performed experiments in the mouse. In this species evidence for the presence of two main subpopulations of lymphocytes, so called "thymus" and "bone marrow-dependent" cells, has recently been obtained [8, 9, 12]. Experiments by various groups have shown that immunologlobulin determinants were primarily present on lymphocytes derived from the bone marrow. Our approach was the following: mouse spleen cells were first incubated with C'-coated red cells (designated EAC)

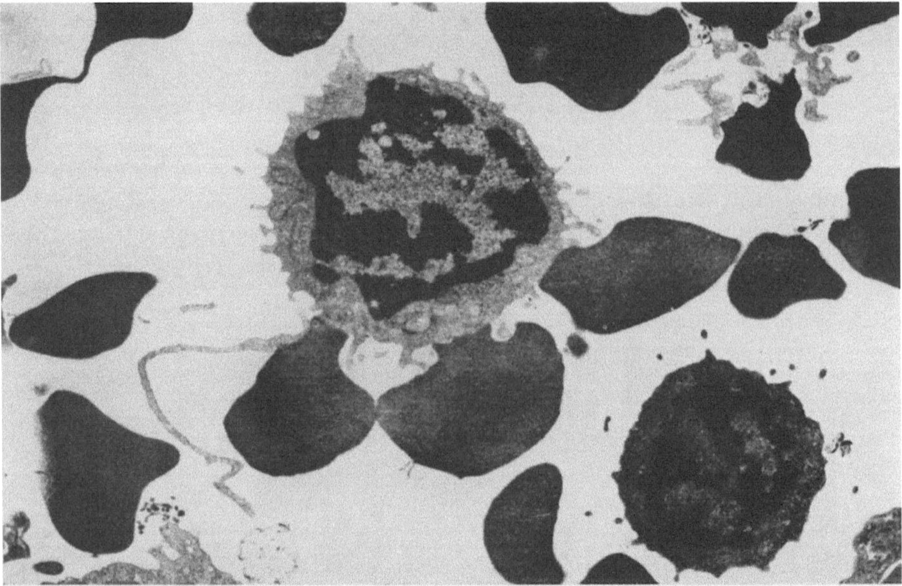

Fig. 2. A receptor positive and a negative blood lymphocyte after incubation with EAC

and then depleted of rosette-forming lymphocytes by centrifugation in a density gradient. In parallel lymphocytes were reacted with EA-sensitized red cells without C- and were then centrifuged similarly. The percentage of lymphocytes with kappa determinants was evaluated in a cytotoxic assay. Consistently, a loss of lymphocytes with receptor sites for antigen-antibody-complement complexes resulted also in a loss of lymphocytes with immunoglobulin determinants as detected with anti-kappa antisera (Table 1). Our observations of a rather close relationship between receptor positive lymphocytes and those with immunoglobulin determinants are in accord

Table 1. *Experiment on the relationship of C receptor positive lymphocytes (CRL) to lymphocytes bearing kappa determinants using mouse spleen cells*

	Viability (%)	CRL (%)	Lymphocytes reacting with anti-kappa antiserum (%) [a]
Control lymphocytes	89	36	34
CRL depleted lymphocytes [b]	81	0	0

[a] Reacting in a cytotoxic assay with anti-kappa antiserum; corrected for dead cells in the blank:

$$\frac{a-b}{c} \times 100$$

a = dead cells in the presence of antiserum and C (%).
b = dead cells in the presence of C without antiserum (blank).
c = viable cells in the blank (%).

[b] Lymphocytes were incubated with EAC (in controls with EA) and rosette forming cells removed by centrifugation in 23%—33% BSA (7000 g; 30'; 4° C).

with recent experiments by NUSSENZWEIG and his group [1]. Preliminary experiments also suggested that simultaneously with a loss of cells with immunoglobulin determinants an enrichment of lymphocytes with antigenic determinants of thymus-derived cells occured [9]. In the mouse a "helper" mechanism for facilitating the interaction of so-called marrow-derived lymphocytes with antigens has been described [12]. Whether the capacity of certain lymphocytes to bind antigens in the presence of antibody and complement provides a further "helper" mechanism requires further investigations.

A group of patients with chronic lymphocytic leukaemia was investigated in terms of their number of blood lymphocytes bearing the C′ receptor (Fig. 3). The

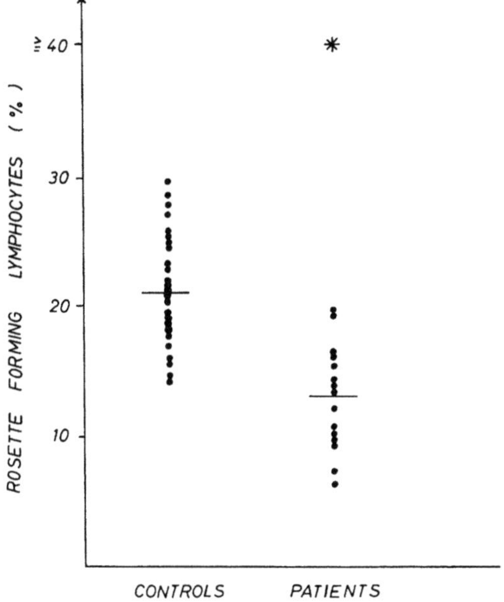

Fig. 3. Percentage of blood lymphocytes forming rosettes with EAC: comparison between normals (25) and patients with chronic lymphocytic leukaemia (16)

group included patients in early and advanced stages of this disease. A reduced percentage of receptor positive lymphocytes was observed in more than half of these patients. One patient, however, consistently showed a very high percentage of receptor positive lymphocytes. This untreated patient presented with severe haematological abnormalities (Hb 5.0%, WBC 202 000/mm³ with 96% lymphocytes, platelets 7 000/mm³), reduced immunoglobulins (γG 435 mg%, γM 35 mg%, γA 108 mg%) and marked splenomegaly.

The number of blood lymphocytes with receptor sites for C′ and those with determinants for kappa chains was compared in some of the patients with chronic lymphocytic leukaemia. The highest percentage of lymphocytes with kappa determinants (21—38%) was observed in the patient with the largest number of lymphocytes with C' receptors. Two patients of our series with a low portion of lymphocytes with C' receptors (7%, 8%) also showed a small percentage of lymphocytes with these immunoglobulin determinants (less than 1%, 2.5%). Three other patients exhibited intermediate values (4—18%).

Chronic lymphocytic leukaemia represents a disease with marked variability in clinical features, concomitant immunological abnormalities and response to treatment. A single patient with a high percentage of lymphocytes reacting with anti-kappa as well as anti-μ antisera has recently been reported by JOHANNSON and KLEIN [5]. The evaluation of lymphocytes with membrane receptors for antigen-antibody-C' complexes apparently provides a simple test system for further studies of the heterogeneity of this disease.

In conclusion: around 20% of normal human blood lymphocytes showed receptor activity for antigen-antibody-C' complexes, some interacting very intimately with the lymphocyte membrane. In the mouse these cells appeared related to marrow-derived lymphocytes. Suggestive evidence for some relationship between these cells and those with immunoglobulin determinants as evaluated with anti-kappa antisera was also obtained in humans.

Acknowledgements

We thank Dr. H. WIGZELL, Karolinska Institute Stockholm for providing us with the anti-kappa antiserum. The excellent technical assistance of Mrs. F. OBERWASSERLECHNER, Mrs. A. MANESCHG, Mrs. U. MICHLMAYR and Mrs. U. WISCHHAUSEN is gratefully acknowledged.

References

1. BIANCO, C., PATRICK, R., NUSSENZWEIG, V,: J. exp. Med. (in press).
2. COOMBS, R. R. A., FRANKS, D.: Progr. Allergy 13, 174 (1969).
3. Huber, H., FUDENBERG, H. H.: Int. Arch. Allergy 34, 18 (1968).
4. — POLLEY, M. J., LINSCOTT, W. D., FUDENBERG, H. H., MÜLLER-EBERHARD, H. J.: Science 162, 1281 (1968).
5. JOHANNSON, B., KLEIN, E.: Clin. exp. Immun. 6, 421 (1970).
6. LAY, H. W., NUSSENZWEIG, V.: J. exp. Med. 128, 991 (1968).
7. LOBUGLIO, A. F., COTRAN, R. S., JANDL, J. H.: Science 158, 1582 (1967).
8. MILLER, J. F. A. P., MITCHELL, G. F.: J. exp. Med. 128, 801 (1968).
9. RAFF, M. C.: Nature 224, 378 (1969).
10. — STERNBERG, M., TAYLOR, R. B.: Nature 225, 553 (1970).
11. RAIDT, D. J., MISHELL, R. I., DUTTON, R. W.: J. exp. Med. 128, 681 (1968).
12. RAJEWSKY, K., in: Current Problems in Immunology. Eds.: O. WESTPHAL, H. E. BOCK, and E. GRUNDMANN. Berlin-Heidelberg-New York: Springer 1969, p. 91.
13. RIEBER, H. P., RIETHMÜLLER, G.: Paper read at the first session of the Society for Immunology, Freiburg/Brsg., Oct. 16—18 (1969).
14. SELL, S., ASOFSKY, R.: Progr Allergy 12, 86 (1968).

Studies on the Biological Properties of the Isolated Active Fractions of Phytohaemagglutinin (PHA) from Phaseolus vulgaris*

K. Schumacher, G. Wintzer, H. Oerkermann, G. Uhlenbruck, G. Alzer, W. D. Hirschmann, and R. Gross

With 3 Figures

Cell-bound immune reactions, especially those which are concerned with the transformation of lymphocytes to blast cells, attract increasing interest. In spite of numerous investigations, the process of lymphocyte stimulation is not yet understood in detail.

The stimulation of lymphocytes by phytohaemagglutinin (PHA) is a proved model for investigation of the different steps of the lymphocyte reactions [1]. In our study we tried to answer the following two questions:

1. Are the different reactions of lymphocytes after stimulation with PHA caused by only one or more stimulating substances?

2. Is the PHA-specific receptor which was recently isolated from red blood cells [2, 3] identical on erythrocytes and lymphocytes?

To answer these questions it was necessary to isolate the active fractions from PHA and to characterize them in their biological properties. As starting material we used a purified PHA (PHA-P Difco). Agglutination of red blood cells and lymphocytes, and stimulation of lymphocytes to blast cell transformation and cytoaggressiveness in tissue cultures were used as test systems.

First we fractionated PHA-P by gel filtration on Sephadex G 100 with subsequent separation by cation exchange chromatography. After gel filtration we found the agglutinating activity for both red blood cells and lymphocytes in the first peak. In view of the elution volume, a molecular weight of about 130,000 was suggested. But pure fractions could not be obtained in this way. The active fractions contained 5—6 components.

The further fractionation was carried out in the following way: after fractionation of PHA-P by chromatography on SE-Sephadex C 50, according to Weber [4, 5], the active fractions II and III were exhaustively absorbed with porcine red blood cells. The absorption of the fractions was followed by further separation by isoelectric focusing in an ampholine column.

The fractionation of PHA-P by cation exchange chromatography on SE-Sephadex C 50 (Fig. 1) by stepwise elution with buffers of different pH values yielded 3 frac-

* Supported by Deutsche Forschungsgemeinschaft.

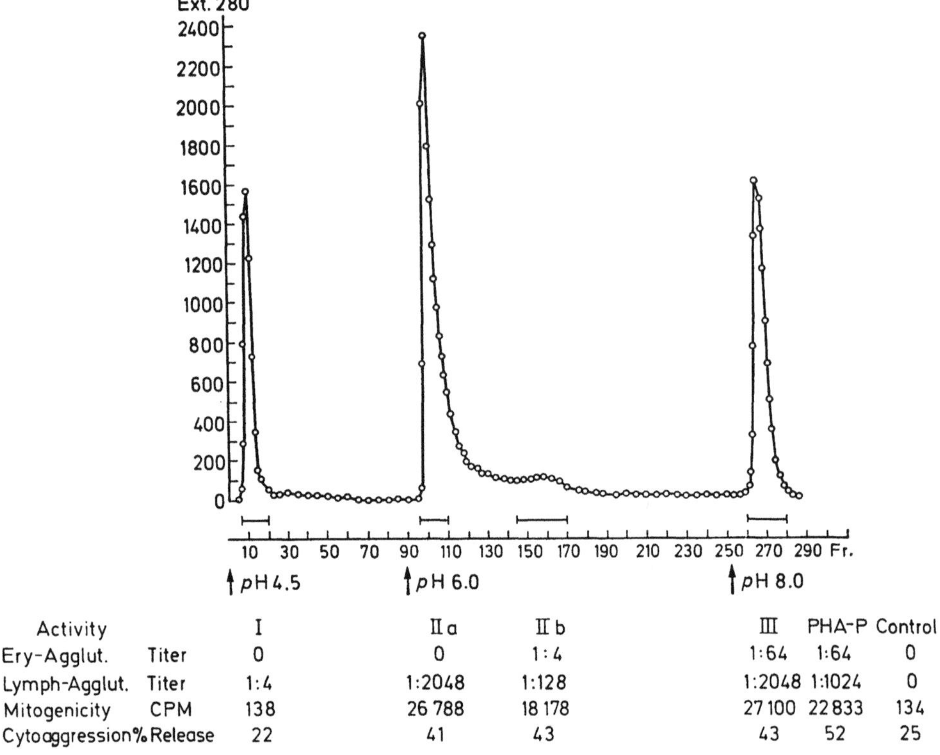

Activity		I	IIa	IIb	III	PHA-P	Control
Ery-Agglut.	Titer	0	0	1:4	1:64	1:64	0
Lymph-Agglut.	Titer	1:4	1:2048	1:128	1:2048	1:1024	0
Mitogenicity	CPM	138	26788	18178	27100	22833	134
Cytoaggression % Release		22	41	43	43	52	25

Fig. 1. Cation exchange chromatography on SE-Sephadex C 50 of PHA-P. Determination of the biological properties of the fractions

tions. Only fractions II and III showed biological activity. Fraction II contained preponderantly the lymphoagglutinating activity, fraction III showed lymphoagglutination as well as erythroagglutination. Further, both fractions had mixed agglutinating, mitogenic and cytoaggressiveness-inducing activity.

Consequently, both fractions showed an immunologic identity reaction with PHA-P and one another. This means, that at least one active substance, the lymphoagglutinin we suppose, must be present in both fractions.

For further purification fraction IIa was exhaustively absorbed with porcine red blood cells to eliminate all erythroagglutinating activity. The absorption was necessary because we had discovered a strong erythroagglutinating activity in this fraction using red blood cells from pig, horse and dove, while human red blood cells were almost not agglutinated.

The absorption procedure was followed by isoelectric focusing of the active fraction (Fig. 2). By this separation 7 fractions could be obtained. The testing of the biological activity of the fractions showed the highest lymphoagglutinating activity in fraction VI, while the strongest mitogenic activity was localized in fraction V. But these differences are significant. Both fractions V and VI were equally potent in inducing cytoaggressive activity of lymphocytes on monolayers in tissue cultures.

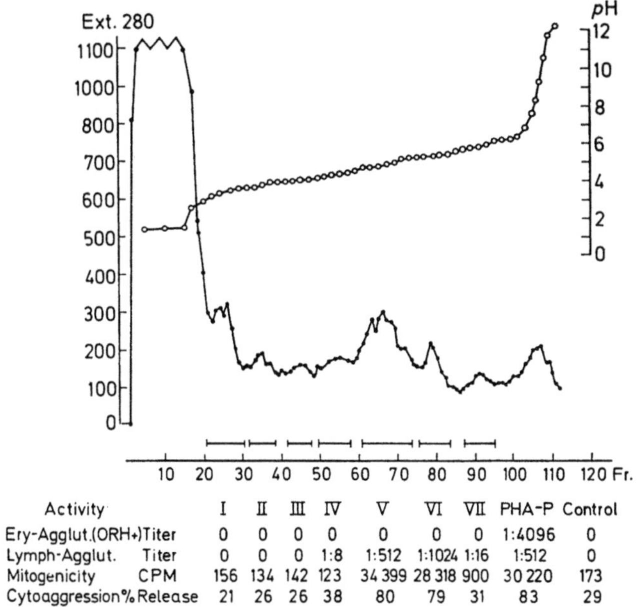

Activity		I	II	III	IV	V	VI	VII	PHA-P	Control
Ery-Agglut.(ORH+)	Titer	0	0	0	0	0	0	0	1:4096	0
Lymph-Agglut.	Titer	0	0	0	1:8	1:512	1:1024	1:16	1:512	0
Mitogenicity	CPM	156	134	142	123	34 399	28 318	900	30 220	173
Cytoaggression % Release		21	26	26	38	80	79	31	83	29

Fig. 2. Fractionation of the lymphoagglutinating fraction from PHA-P by isoelectric focusing. Determination of the biological properties of the fractions

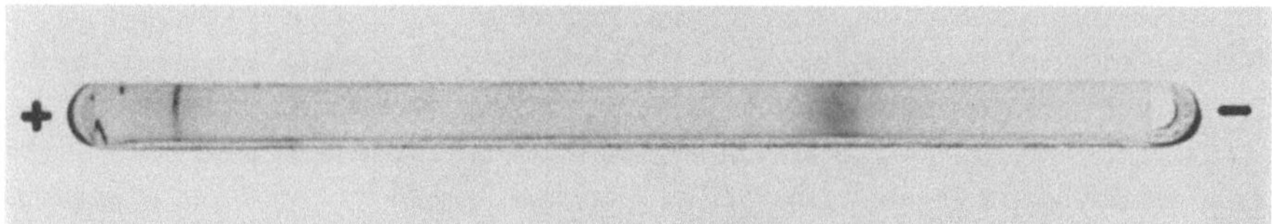

Fig. 3 a. Discelectrophoresis at pH 8.2 of the purified lymphoagglutinin

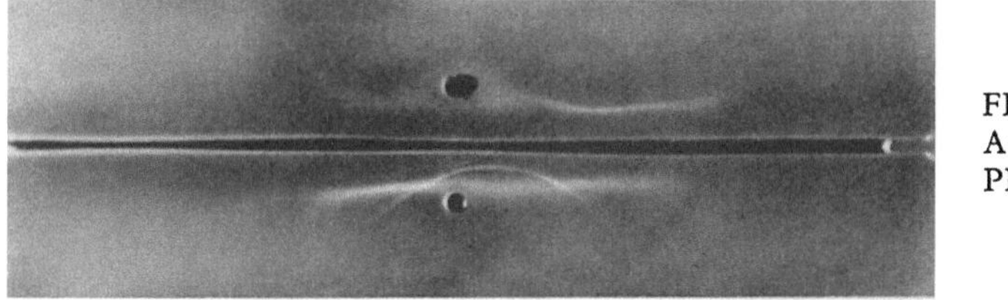

Fig. 3 b. Immunoelectrophoresis at pH 8.6 of PHA-P and the purified lymphoagglutinin. The cathode is to the right. The upper hole contained purified lymphoagglutinin, the lower hole PHA-P. The anti-serum well contained rabbit anti-PHA-P serum

The physico-chemical characterization of the active fractions by discelectrophoresis in polyacrylamide (Fig. 3 a) showed only one component in fraction VI, and two components in fraction V.

By immunoelectrophoresis (Fig. 3 b), developed with a rabbit anti-PHA-P serum, fraction VI gave one precipitation line in the direction of the cathode. This line seems to correspond to the lymphoagglutinin isolated by WEBER [5].

The existence of two fractions with different isoelectric points but identical biological activity indicates, that PHA-P contains two different lymphoagglutinins with very similar physico-chemical properties. This assumption is supported by the finding of different fractions with different isoelectric points after re-focusing of the isolated fractions V and VI.

In spite of the slight physico-chemical differences, these two fractions showed almost identical biological properties. The differences of the fractions, concerning lymphoagglutination, mitogenicity and induction of cytoaggressiveness are very small.

Further, it was impossible to infer or assign single biological properties to different sites on the active molecule. By periodate treatment (0.1 M) the lympho-agglutinating as well as the mitogenic and cytoaggressiv effect of the purified substance was destroyed.

In agreement with other authors [6, 7, 8, 9, 10, 11], we found that the separation of the lymphocyte stimulating and agglutinating activity from the erythroagglutinating factor was possible. However, the inhibition tests produced less clear results. In most experiments the lymphoagglutinating titre was reduced by absorption with red blood cells. Otherwise the erythroagglutination titre was reduced by absorption with lymphocytes. But the lymphoagglutinating activity could be eliminated by red blood cell absorption.

On the other hand, we found striking differences between erythroagglutination and lymphoagglutination by inhibition tests, which were carried out with the isolated PHA-specific receptor from porcine red blood cells. The erythroagglutination was completely inhibited by "mucoid" (Uhlenbruck [2]) while lymphoagglutination and stimulation to mitogenicity and cytoaggressiveness were not inhibited.

From these results we suppose, that the PHA-specific receptor on red blood cells is not identical with the receptor on lymphocytes. On the other hand, the phenomenon of mixed agglutination by the purified lymphoagglutinin suggests that red blood cells may also carry the lymphocyte receptor, or parts of it, in small amounts.

This problem will be discussed in the following paper.

References

1. Naspitz, Ch. K., Richter, M.: Progr. Allergy 12, 185 (1968).
2. Uhlenbruck, G., Reifenberg, U., Oyen, R.: Z. Naturforsch. 24 b (1969).
3. Kornfeld, St., Kornfeld, R.: Proc. nat. Acad. Sci. (Wash.) 63, 1439 (1969).
4. Weber, Th. H., Nordman, C. T., Gräsbeck, R.: Scand. J. Haemat. 4, 77 (1967).
5. — Scand. J. clin. Lab. Invest. 24, Suppl. 111, 1—80 (1969).
6. Rigas, D. A., Johnson, E. A.: Ann. N.Y. Acad. Sci. 113, 800 (1964).
7. Holland, N. H., Holland, P.: Nature (Lond.) 207, 1307 (1965).
8. Barkhan, P., Ballas, A.: Nature (Lond.) 200, 141 (1963).
9. Kolodny, R. L., Hirschhorn, K.: Nature (Lond.) 201, 715 (1964).
10. Nordman, C. T., de la Chapelle, A., Gräsbeck, R.: Acta med. scand. Suppl. 412, 49 (1964).
11. Rigas, D. A., Head, Ch.: Biochem. biophys. Res. Comm. 34, 633 (1969).

The Nature of the PHA Receptor on Red Cells

G. Uhlenbruck, G. Wintzer, K. Schumacher, H. Oerkermann, G. I. Pardoe, W. D. Hirschmann, G. Alzer, and R. Gross

With 3 Figures

In 1969, we found [1], that the so-called PHA (*Phaseolus vulgaris*) receptor for red cell agglutination was located in the glycoprotein fraction of the outer red cell membrane. This could be demonstrated by immunodiffusion in agargel, where a mucoid preparation from pig red cells precipitated with PHA from *Phaseolus vulgaris* DIFCO, in a similar way to own preparation from wax bean, both giving an identity line with the red cell mucoid.

We isolated this receptor by phenol/saline extraction from the genuine stroma and submitted the underlayer with the glycoproteins to isoelectric focusing. As a result of our experiments, we found that the glycoproteins obtained in that way can be divided into two groups: neuraminic acid (NA) containing and NA free glycoproteins and even pure proteins. This is shown in Fig. 1, where also the PHA activity

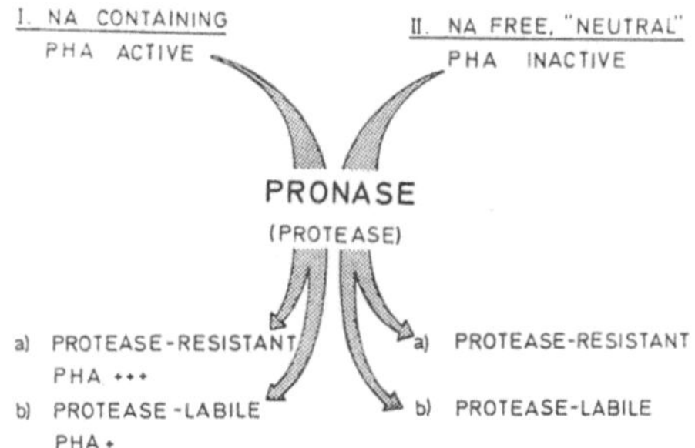

Fig. 1. Red cell glycoproteins (Phenol/saline) and PHA activity

of these fractions is given: in this connection, it is very interesting that the PHA activity seems to be associated with the NA-containing fraction and especially that it remains after protease treatment on the protease-resistant part on the membrane. This conclusion was mainly drawn from agglutination studies with normal and enzyme-treated cells (Table 1). After pronase treatment we found always an increase of the titer, usually more than after neuraminidase treatment. The latter fact may be due either to uncovering of new sites or to the incomplete behaviour of the agglu-

Table 1. *Agglutination of different rbc by PHA*

Red blood cells	Normal	Pronase-treated	RDE-treated
Pig	64,000	500,000	500,000
Human	2,000	500,000	128,000
Cat	64,000	64,000	64,000
Duck	1,000	64,000	512
Rabbit	8,000	16,000	16,000
Pigeon	8,000	16,000	16,000
Dog	2,000	4,000	512
Chicken	4	2,000	32
Horse	256	128	512
Bovine	0	32,000	0

tinin. It is interesting that with bovine red cells, the receptor for PHA is serologically detectable after pronase treatment only. This is interpreted by us as the inactivity of

$$\text{Gal} \xrightarrow[\beta]{1 \rightarrow 4} \text{GNAc} \rightarrow \quad \text{or} \quad \text{Gal} \xrightarrow[\beta]{1 \rightarrow 3} \text{GNAc} \rightarrow$$

structures to serve as PHA receptors, because those structures arise especially after neuraminidase treatment of bovine red cells. This is in full agreement with Korn-feld's [2] findings, that a third sugar—D-mannose—is an essential part of the PHA receptor. Accordingly we can conclude that these mannose-containing structures are located in the keeper clefts of the membrane and belong to the protease-resistant glycoprotein skeleton. Also in inhibition studies we found, that N-Acetyl-Lactos-amine (Gal $\xrightarrow[\beta]{1 \rightarrow 4}$ GNAc) containing glycoproteins without mannose did not inhibit the PHA agglutination. On the other side, especially in bovine red cells, N-acetyl-lactosamine is well detected by the lectin from *Ricinus communis* and anti-Pneumococcus-Type-XIV antisera. In other words: both these agglutinins react with the lactosamine part of the PHA receptor, but on the other hand, are not capable of transforming lymphocytes. If, however, the red cell agglutination receptor and the one for mitogenic action are identical, it seems that for the latter an agglutinin with a larger combining side including mannose or even more [2] is necessary. This could explain why certain antilymphocytic reagents are mitogenic, and others not. Furthermore, we assume that a certain distance between the receptors on the cell is essential, either because one agglutinin bound to two receptors, or two agglutinins reacting with neighbouring receptors and held together by a "mitogenic principle" may induce the transformation by an allosteric effect in distortion of the membrane surface.

In Fig. 2 the result of an isoelectric focusing is represented. PHA inhibition activity is in the region of the NA-containing glycoproteins, whereas the other fractions have no activity. The method is fully described elsewhere [3]. Furthermore, the heterogeneity of these red cell mucoids is remarkable, as shown by the different "isoelectric" peaks. A similar heterogeneity is revealed in the protease-labile fraction, which has less PHA activity because of the breakdown of the protein backbone, and is modified when different enzymes are used. The same holds for blood from individual animals, which all have their characteristic "isoelectric" glycoprotein

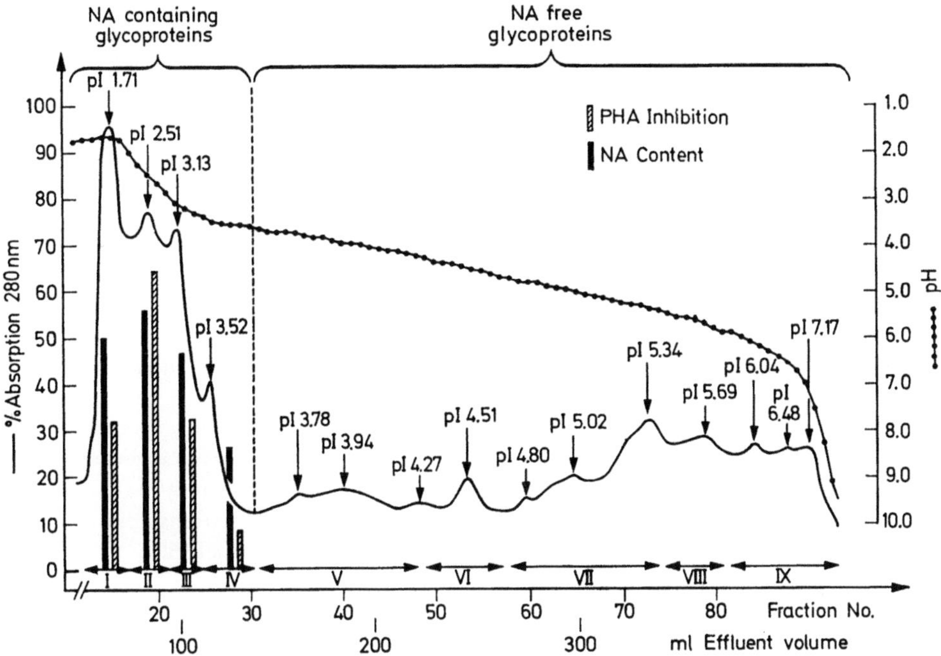

Fig. 2. Isoelectric focusing of pig red cell glycoprotein fraction

pattern (unpublished results). Also the PHA activity is always present in several NA-containing glycoprotein fractions.

In testing the PHA activity of these and other substances, we found that it is also important which "indicator" cell is used in the haemagglutination inhibiton system. We can (for what reason we don't exactly know, maybe the numbers of receptors are essential, or the protein backbone near the carbohydrate receptor, or its steric environment) distinguish between strong and weak receptors either on the cell or on the inhibitor, as outlined in the scheme in Fig. 3. We made the interesting observation that it is possible to convert strong receptor rbc into weak receptor rbc by pronase treatment, although the titer with PHA may even be increased, thus while the cell appears to have a stronger affinity for the agglutinin, the reverse is the case:

$$\text{strong receptor pig rbc} \xrightarrow{\text{Pronase}} \text{weak receptor pig rbc}$$
$$\text{(titer 64.000)} \qquad \text{(titer 500.000)}$$

For instance, in the first case the inhibiton titer calculated to 8 AD when using pig rbc mucoid as inhibitor was 16, in the second case 128.

Good inhibition is obtained with either strong or weak receptors on both reactants, particle-bound or soluble. The inhibition is weak when the competition between the agglutinin and both these receptors is won by the cellular receptor, when the soluble inhibitor is relatively weak with regard to the cell-bound one. This

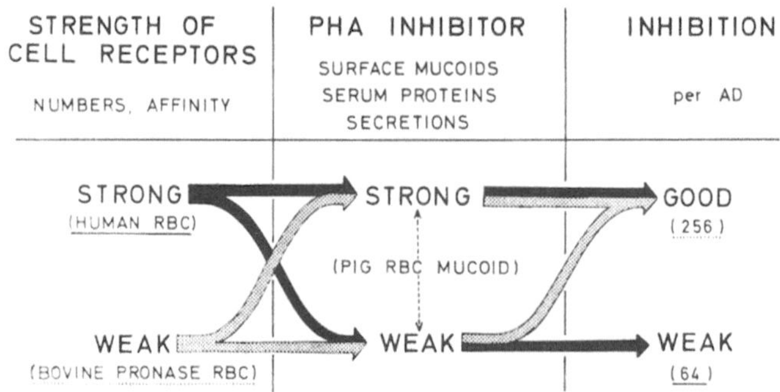

Fig. 3. Competitive inhibition studies in the PHA receptor system (cell-bound soluble inhibitor, bound receptor)

method elucidates also the problem of the "receptor side" which may be influenced by several factors (allosteric, environment, affinity, spatial relationships), so that "new" properties like mitogenicity may arise from an agglutinin molecule.

Summary

The method of isoelectric focusing was applied to pig red cell glycoproteins, to demonstrate the heterogeneity of the erythroagglutinin receptor for the lectin from *Phaseolus vulgaris*. The receptor activity was found only in the neuraminic acid containing fractions and not in the neutral glycoprotein material. In this connection competitive inhibition studies with normal and enzyme-treated red cells and various inhibitors are discussed.

References

1. Uhlenbruck, G., Reifenberg, U., Oyen, R.: Z. Naturforsch. 24 b, 224 (1969).
2. Kornfeld, R., Kornfeld, S.: J. biol. Chem. 245, 2536—2545 (1970).
3. Wintzer, G., Uhlenbruck, G.: Z. Physiol. Chem. 351, 834—838 (1970).

Immunochemistry of Galactosyl Groups
of Cell Membranes

G. I. Pardoe, G. W. G. Bird, G. Uhlenbruck, and D. J. Anstee

With 4 Figures

Carbohydrates play an important role in cell surface antigens: these are present in cell surfaces not as large aggregates (polysaccharide) but in relatively short chains comprising hexoses and hexosamines, attached to proteins or lipids functioning as carrier molecules. Moreover, the point of attachment to cell surface proteins has so far been shown to be either between β-D-GpNAc and asparagine or α-D-GalpNAc and a hydroxyamino (serine or threonine) side chains, with a possible slight bias towards threonine. These two types of linkage differ in their reaction with alkali, the former being resistant and the latter highly susceptible to pH above 8.0. Glycolipids have a ceramido structure carrying either β-D-Gp or β-D-Galp in glycosidic linkage. These various structures are illustrated in Figure 1. With the exception of one type of glycolipid, galactosyl groups are not directly attached to the non-sugar aglycone (carrier or acceptor molecule).

Sugar units are transferred from specific nucleotide donors to the growing carbohydrate chain; specific glycosyl transferases mediate the reaction and the site to which the new sugar is attached to the acceptor sugar unit is higly characteristic for the transferase; this enzyme is also selective with respect to the penultimate sugar, and environment (protein or lipid, hydrophilic or hydrophobic) of the acceptor [6]. Galactosyl groups in cell surface components are only known to be transferred to N-acetyl-hexosamine or other galactosyl groups, and not directly to mannosyl groups; there is a whole family of galactosyl transferases utilising the same donor (UDP-Gal) but different acceptors (Fig. 2 a and b). Some transferases specifically add β-galactosyl units; other add α-galactosyl groups, and the products are associated with blood group B specificity; β-galactosyl groups added to an alkali-sensitive glycopeptide linkage are associated with blood group M, N specificity [6, 9]. The acceptor substrates themselves arise by stepwise addition of sugars and in each case, the sequence of these is governed by a linked enzyme system,—the Multi-Glycosyl-Transferase (MGT) system of Roseman [10, 11]. The various substrates themselves arise because of the influence of the different transferases and there is a degree of randomness in these syntheses because the kinetics of the different systems vary, so that truncated chains at all points may be present as normal cell surface components. In glycoprotein biosynthesis, galactosyl groups are added within the cell at the cytoplasmic level although the initial hexosamine-addition step appears to take place on the ribosomes [1].

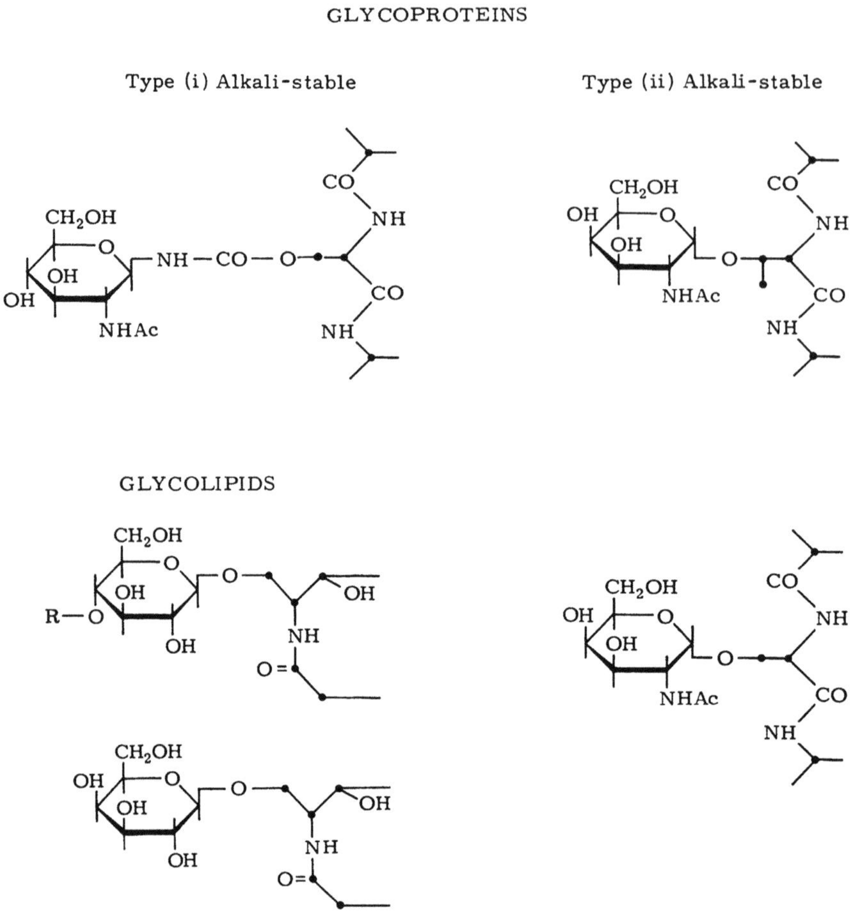

GLYCOPROTEINS

Type (i) Alkali-stable   Type (ii) Alkali-stable

GLYCOLIPIDS

Fig. 1. Primary structures of glycopeptide and glycolipid linkages in cell surfaces

How then do galactosyl units occur in the cell surface? They are synthesised in
the cell; carbohydrate synthesis is subsequent to polypeptide chain synthesis and the
location of the carbohydrate chains depends upon the acceptor amino acid on the
ribosomal growing peptide chain being in a favourable conformation to accept the
donor hexosamine. Other units are added in sequence by the operation of the MGT
system after release of the incomplete glycopeptide into the cytoplasm, and galactosyl
groups are almost the last to be added before export of the total polypeptide (probably *via* the Golgi apparatus); immediately the polypeptide is exported, it is
organised into the appropriate tertiary structure by tight binding between lipids and
its own α-helical hydrophobic structure, characteristic of membrane structural
protein. The hydrophilic areas with associated heterosaccharide chains are peripher-
ally oriented; ZAHLER [15] has an excellent model of this concept (Fig. 3) and for
our purpose, the galactosyl groups may be located in the hydrophilic "cap", which
we visualise as a tertiary folded polypeptide chain having numerous heterosaccharide

β-GALACTOSYL ACCEPTORS

(2 transferases, one for
seryl-and one for
threonyl-)

Fig. 2 a

α-GALACTOSYL ACCEPTORS

Blood group B determinants

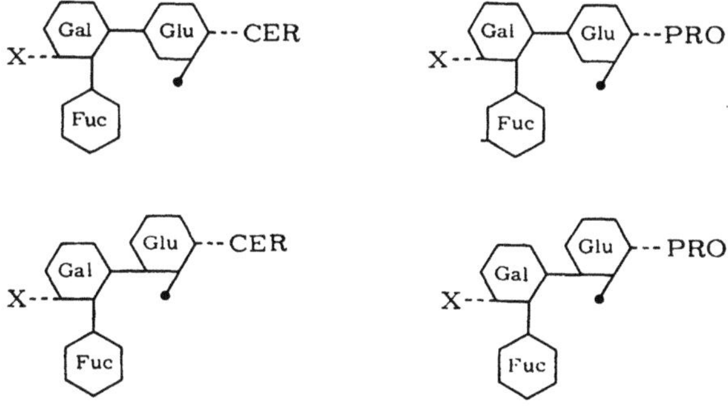

Fig. 2 b

Fig. 2 a and b. Substrates for specific galactosyl transferases, present in cell surface structures

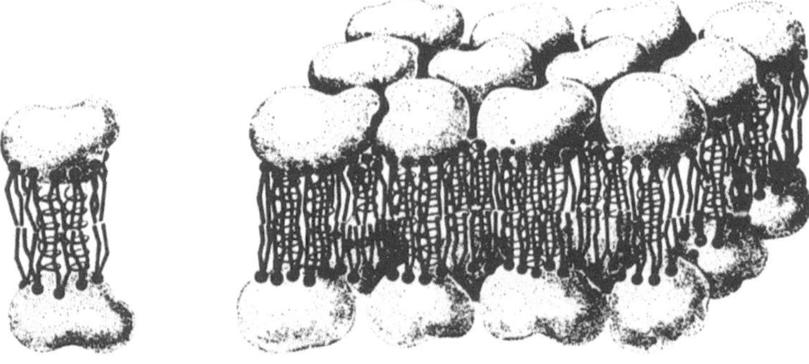

Fig. 3. Cell surface organisation. (After P. Zahler [15])

chains which are normally disposed to the surface, as well as in the "heads" of the glycolipids, tightly bound by α-helical protein and shielded by the overhanging hydrophilic "cap". Thus, galactosyl groups are associated with both glycolipid and glycoprotein carriers, and some of the latter may also be associated with hydrophobic regions of the cell surface, characteristically resistant to the action of proteases, as indicated in Table 1. Proteases remove the hydrophilic glycopeptide "cap"

Table 1. *Distribution of galactosyl groups between hydrophilic and hydrophobic regions of the cell surface*

Cells	Hydrophilic Glycoprotein	Hydrophobic Glycoprotein	Glycolipid
Untreated	$+++$	$+$	$+$
Protease-RDE-	$(+)$ or $\emptyset$ unchanged or enhanced	$+++$ unchanged	$+++$ unchanged or enhanced

from the cell surface, exposing the hidden crypt-antigens [12, 14]. The protease selected should have broad specificity: the surface glycoprotein obtained by phenol-saline extraction of red cell stroma mass is deficient in aromatic amino acids and in cystine, so that in general the chymotrypsins are less effective than trypsin (which cleaves at the well-represented basic amino acids) and the thiol-activated plant proteases behave as broad-spectrum proteases irrespective of their active thiol groups. In Fig. 4 is illustrated our concept of the relative sites of separation using proteases or phenol-saline extraction procedures. The major difference between the glycoprotein extracted by phenol-saline rom stroma mass and the glycopeptides separated by protease treatment lies in the increased content of hydrophobic amino acids in the former [6]. All the proteases seem to cleave at a susceptible region somewhere near the hydrophobic peptide chains. In all cases, the carbohydrate units appear unaffected by the extraction or separation procedure used, so that these separated fragments may be used as specific inhibitory substances for investigating cell surface

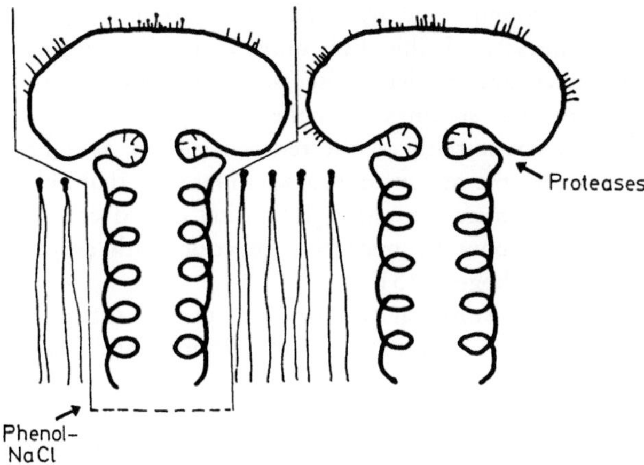

Fig. 4. Cell surface structure showing sites of action of proteases and of phenol-saline extraction

sugar determinants in serological procedures. At the outset, we stressed the significance of carbohydrates in cell surface antigens (defining antigens as units binding antisera) and the frequently-occurring terminal galactosyl groups are especially important. A new dimension has been added to methods of elucidating the structure of the determinants of the intact cell surface by the use of heterophile agglutinins, derived from such exotic sources as seeds, fungi, molluscs, invertebrate hemolymph and fish ova. Our groups have been investigating and defining the specificities of these various proteins, which bind to a single sugar unit, or even a part of a pyranose ring, to that these reagents can serve to elucidate the specificity of antigen-antibody reactions. In Table 2 is a classification of heterophile agglutinins having specificity for D-galactosyl groups; some of these reagents can differentiate between α- and β-linked galactosyl group (e. g. *Fomes fomentarius* and *Ricinus communis*); others

Table 2. *Heterophile agglutinins binding galactosyl groups*

α-β-D-Galp-	α-D-Galp-	β-D-Galp-
Evonymus europaeus (?)	*Evonymus europaeus*	*Amaranthus caudatus*
Ricinus communis	*Fomes fomentarius*	*Arachis hypogoea*
Sophora japonica	*Clupea harangus*	*Bauhinia purpurea*
Anti-S.XIV antisera	*Salmo irideus*	*Maclura aurantica*
	Salmo salar	*Phaseolus vulgaris*
		Ricinus communis
		Soja hispida
		Vicia graminea
		Viscum album
		Wistaria sinensis
		Anti-T (T-agglutinin)

distinguish between hydrophilic and hydrophobic locations (e. g. *Maclura aurantica* and *Amaranthus caudatus*); of this list, only *Phaseolus vulgaris* has mitogenic activity for lymphocytes, and we have discussed this elsewhere in this Symposium. *Arachis hypogoea* also binds specifically in the hydrophilic region: in this case, the galactosyl group is present initially in the red cell surface as a Friedenreich crypt-antigen, revealed only by the action of neuraminidase, so that this agglutinin is an excellent reagent for demonstrating panagglutination of red cells as a result of "T-transformation" brought about by microbial infection with associated neuraminidase biosynthesis by the pathogen [13].

It is also possible to distinguish the locations of cell surface blood group and other carbohydrate receptors (Table 3) and the differentiation between hydrophilic (protease-labile) and hydrophobic (protease-resistant) regions provides a rapid routine diagnostic approach. The determinants of the M, N and related and satellite systems are associated with the hydrophilic region and are highly dependent upon neuraminyl end-groups (associated also with galactosyl carriers) for their specificity [9, 12] whereas the galactosyldependent B receptors (and associated A, H antigens) as well as the P, Ii systems are all associated with the hydrophobic regions.

Table 3. *Distribution of blood group and other carbohydrate cell surface receptors between hydrophilic and hydrophobic regions of the erythrocyte*

	Hydrophilic protein	protein		Hydrophobic lipid
Blood group determinants	M, N and related systems	P		A, B, H
	S, s, U	I, i		Lewis (Acquired)
	Duffy		Rhesus	P
	Tn		Cad	I, i
Surface receptors	Myxoviral Mononucleosis Lipopolysaccharide Pr; Sp; M^{duc} *Phaseolus vulgaris* *Ricinus communis*	Myxoviral *Phaseolus vulgaris* *Ricinus communis*		*Ricinus communis*

Whe have therefore a means of handling intact cells, available in small numbers, by methods which will give precise information of the immunochemistry of their antigens without causing irrevocable cell damage (and so obviating false results from contamination with intracellular components). We have adapted these methods to look at other cell types, notably lymphoid cells. We used Burkitt EB2 lymphoma cells [4, 5] because these can initiate blast transformation by normal lymphocytes. By differential absorption before and after treatment with protease, we have demonstrated the distribution of galactosyl groups in these cells in the hydrophobic and hydrophilic regions, and have shown the absence of typical M- and N-like and "T-" antigens. Some of the galactosyl receptors in these cells are listed in Table 4. It is interesting that in the Burkitt EB2 cells, the carbohydrate-receptor for *Phaseolus*

Table 4. *Galactosyl receptors detected in Burkitt EB2 lymphoma cells*

	Untreated	Protease-	RDE-
Amaranthus caudatus	+ + +	⌀	n. d.
Arachis hypogoea	⌀	⌀	⌀
Bauhinia purpurea	⌀	⌀	n. d.
Maclura aurantica	+ + +	+ + +	n. d.
Molucella laevis	+ + +	+ + +	n. d.
Phaseolus vulgaris	+ + +	⌀	n. d.
Ricinus communis	+ + +	+ + +	+ + +
Vicia graminea	⌀	⌀	n. d.
Viscum album	+ + +	⌀	n. d.
Wistaria sinensis	⌀	⌀	n. d.
Rabbit anti-M	⌀	⌀	n. d.
Rabbit anti-N	⌀	⌀	n. d.

vulgaris is removed by protease-treatment. This work is our approach to the investigation of the immunochemistry of carbohydrate groups of the surfaces of intact viable cells. We use specific proteases and glycosidase; heterophile agglutinins and antibodies of defined specificity. These reagents enable us to obviate many artefacts arising during manipulation of cell extracts, and are valuable rapid diagnostic tools.

Resume

Cell surface antigens involving immunodominant groups are distributed in hydrophilic and hydrophobic regions of cell surfaces; they are associated with peptide and lipid carriers. They may be detected using specific heterophile agglutinins before or after treating intact viable cells with enzymes of defined specificity. In erythrocytes and Burkitt EB2 lymphoma cells, galactosyl determinants are found in hydrophilic and hydrophobic environments.

Abbreviations Used

Formula for sugars are abbreviated as prescribed in the Handbook for Chemical Society Authors (Chemical Society, London 1961). D = dextro; p = pyranose form; G = glucose; Gal = galactose; NANc = acetyl.

In diagrams illustrating structures in Fig. 2 a and b, a simple hexagon is used to show the heterocyclic hexose ring; these are graphic only and are not to be confused with the aromatic benzene ring.

Acknowledgements

This work was carried out using founds provided by the Birmingham and Bristol Regional Hospital Boards and the Deutsche Forschungsgemeinschaft.

References

1. Melchers, F.: Biochemistry 8, 938 (1969).
2. Pardoe, G. I., Bird, G. W. G., Uhlenbruck, G.: Z. Immun.-Forsch. 137, 442 (1969).
3. — — — Sprenger, I., Heggen, M.: Z. Immun.-Forsch. (1970) in press.
4. — Uhlenbruck, G., in: Organtransplantation. Hrsg.: A. Heymer u. D. Ricken. Stuttgart: Schattauer 1969, S. 47.
5. — — J. med. Lab. Technol. 27, 249 (1970).
6. — — J. med. Lab. Technol. (1970) in press.
7. — — Anstee, D. J., Reifenberg, U.: Z. Immun.-Forsch. 139, 468 (1970).
8. — — Bird, G. W. G.: Immunology 18, 73 (1970).
9. — — Reifenberg, U.: J. med. Lab. Technol. (1970) in press.
10. Roseman, S.: Proc. 4th Internat. Congress Cystic Fibrosis, Part II. Basel: Karger 1968, p. 244.
11. — Chem. and Phiysics of Sphingolipids. Ed.: C. C. Sweeley. Amsterdam: North-Holland Publ. Co. 1970 (in press).
12. Uhlenbruck, G., Pardoe, G. I.: Fortschritte der Hämatologie, Bd. 1. Hrsg.: E. Perlick, W. Plenert u. O. Prokop. Leipzig: J. A. Barth VEB 1970, S. 551.
13. — — Bird, G. W. G.: Z. Immun.-Forsch. 138, 423 (1969).
14. — Rothe, A., Pardoe, G. I.: Z. Immun.-Forsch. 136, 79 (1968).
15. Zahler, P.: Experientia 25, 449 (1969).

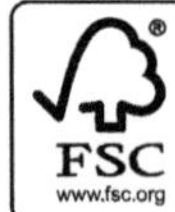

MIX
Papier aus verantwortungsvollen Quellen
Paper from responsible sources
FSC® C105338

If you have any concerns about our products,
you can contact us on
ProductSafety@springernature.com

In case Publisher is established outside the EU,
the EU authorized representative is:
Springer Nature Customer Service Center GmbH
Europaplatz 3, 69115 Heidelberg, Germany

Printed by Libri Plureos GmbH
in Hamburg, Germany